The Essence of Life & Phenomena of Healing
How to heal yourself and others

Cindy Walker

DEDICATION

For Love.

CONTENTS

1 THE SCIENCE OF MENTAL HEALING

Throughout these pages I shall give you the essence and substance of the best scientific knowledge regarding the prevention and cure of physical ailments using the power of the mind.

Mental Healing is a science, not superstition; it is based on scientific facts, not vague imaginings. My goal is to present the information of Mental Healing to you avoiding reference to mysticism or occultism, or strange metaphysical and philosophical theories.

Nature surely contains enough wonders for us, without the need of our exploring any so called supernatural realms in our search for the relief of aches, pains and disease. There is no need for us to become "spooky" or uncanny when we begin the study of Mental Healing, nor when we carry the theory into the realm of actual practice. There are greater wonders and mysteries wrapped up in the domain of Nature than have ever been dreamed of by man in his search of the supernatural.

There is also no need to drag the religious element into Mental Healing, for it has no direct connection with the scientific side of the subject. There is no one who has a greater, deeper, or more profound respect, veneration and reverence than I have for the Power of Nature as shown in all of her activities. I firmly believe that having a strong faith in that Power has an uplifting effect upon the minds and souls of people, and this faith tends to keep them in good health, and also restores health when it is lost. But, I do believe that theology and Mental Healing are two very distinct fields of human thought and activity. I do not believe in making a religion of Mental Healing, and of mixing theological doctrines with the scientific methods of applying it.

In fact, many people have received benefit from Mental Healing administered under the guise and form of religious teaching, I also believe that many more have been repelled and kept away from the wonderful benefits of this form of treatment because of the strange and queer theological teachings of some healers. There is no reason in the world why any person should abandon his or her chosen religion - that faith that has been of great comfort and consolation to him or her during their life - in order to obtain the benefits of "new" healing methods. Rather I do believe that the best therapeutic methods of Mental Healing may be applied with greater results when the patient is supported by the comforting assurance of his or her own chosen faith.

Under the guise of Mental Healing many people have been forced to abandon the faith they grew up with leaving them floating in a sea of unknowing. These people have let go of the old without getting a firm grip on the new.

All religion may be summed up in three general principals

(1) Belief in the existence of a Supreme Being or Power, from whom all life proceeds
(2) faith in, and dependence upon the goodness of that Being or Power in all the affairs and circumstances of daily life
(3) living the "Right Life" in accord with the highest teachings of the best faiths, and in accordance with the dictates of one's own conscience.

Having these principals and living up to them as closely as one can, one is truly religious, no matter what his faith or profession.

So in this understanding you will not be torn away from the safe anchorage of your religious faith, nor asked to accept strange and new theology as a precedent to your learning the art and science of healing yourself and others. While all thinking men recognize the presence and being of a Supreme Power, and seek assistance from it, and depend upon it accordingly; we shall find that this Supreme Power has placed within our reach the means and methods to allow us to study and practice this science, as we would any other science. Mental Healing is neither a religion, nor a theology; it is a scientific system of healing by natural means and methods.

Although the Mind is the great force and power with which cures are made using Mental Healing, we will not be asked to accept any particular metaphysical theory of "what is Mind?" and why should we? Because we do not insist the teachers of physical science explain to us exactly what Matter is! The truth is they do not know; and neither does anyone else. So likewise no one knows just exactly what Mind is; nor are they likely to know. Mind, Matter, and Energy – these are the three great manifestations of the Infinite and Eternal Supreme Power.

But, even though we do not know exactly what Mind is, we do know how it works. Like electricity (something we do not know or understand fully either) we have harnessed Mind to do work for us. We have in Mind a wonderful and potent force of natural energy. We have learned how to guide, direct and apply its energies and power in the direction of healing disease. We have discovered that Mind works as regularly as electricity and we know that we may set it to work in special direction when we provide the channels or programming for its expression.

As we proceed with these lessons, we shall discover that not only does Mind prevent and cure diseases, but that it also causes diseases. Fear has slain more human beings than most disease. Its victims are numbered by the millions. And not only does it kill, but it cripples and incapacitates millions, and renders them miserable and unable to live normal lives, unable to perform efficient work for themselves and those dependent upon them. Like all other great forces, Mind acts negatively as well as positively – it harms as well as heals. Wisdom consists of learning its laws and principals of operation and learning to prevent its undesirable working, to encourage, cultivate and direct its positive, beneficial activities.

With these lessons I will do my best to bring order out of chaos in mental healing. There has been so much misunderstood teaching on the subject and so much fanciful and often absurd theorizing that the intelligent student is often perplexed when he begins studying the subject.

Past teaching regarding the influence of the Mind upon the body has been clouded and distorted by the errors of superstition, the inaccuracies of ignorance, and the exaggeration of fanatical extremists whose prejudiced observations and reports were more or less colored by commercial motives or monetary enthusiasm. So it is no wonder that teaching mental healing grew into a mass of religious contradictions, unreliable observations and groundless assertions. It has required much painstaking labor on the part of modern physiologists and psychologists to clear away the accumulation of rubbish and ignorance, and to lay a scientific foundation for a rational system of mental hygiene based upon the known laws of Mind and Matter.

You will notice in these lessons that I have not confined myself solely to the psychology of Mental Healing. I have accepted the facts of modern physiology as correct and have directed the use of the power of the mind along the lines of these physiological facts. One of the great mistakes of unscientific practitioners of mental healing has been the fact that they have refused to accept physiology as existent; but have used the Mind in a general hit or miss fashion. The scientific practitioner acquaints himself with the physiology of the normal person, and then bends the mental energies toward restoring this normal state and condition of functioning. Knowing how the organs of the body function in health, the practitioner is better able to picture in the mind of the patient (and in his own mind) exactly what conditions are desired to be created. This mental picture is the pattern around which Mind creates, it will be seen that the importance of creating the right kind of mental pattern cannot be overestimated.

In order to understand these lessons completely we will need to understand basic physiology in connection with the psychology of cure. Whenever possible the technical terms will be discarded and when it is impossible to proceed without them we shall explain them in simple terms so everyone will be able to understand them. True knowledge does not consist of a parrot like memorizing or repetition of long words or foreign terms, it consists of an understanding of the real meaning of the things described.

At this time I would like to ask you to set aside all preconceived ideas and acquired prejudices. I don't expect you to accept my theories and methods in preference to your own but rater encourage you to cultivate an open mind to what I have to say until you are able to grasp the why and how of it all. In some cases you may think that I mean something quite different from my real meaning, this is because I may be using different terms than you are used to. We all have our own terms, and we are suspicious of new ones. So we should always be sure that we really understand the true meaning of the terms used by others.

Finally, we must once and for all get rid of the idea that Truth is the exclusive possession of any one school of thought or practice. There is a little good in almost all schools and methods. The most good is always obtained by analyzing the different theories and methods and then taking the essence of all that is best and discarding the rest. This is known as the "eclectic method." Combining the best of the many forms and phases examined, selecting the best in each, and combining this into one general system and method. Any other plan results in narrowness and bigotry, both unscientific and quite contrary to common sense.

Now that we are all the same page, let's begin!

2 THE CORPOREAL MIND

The human body is not a mass of mindless matter. It is an organ of the Mind as is the brain, although its mental work is along different lines. This may seem like a startling statement to the person who has not acquainted himself with the discoveries of modern psychology and physiology.

Not only is the body as a whole the outward expression of an inward mentality, but every part of it (even the cells themselves) have a mind within and acting through it. Every part has its own mental being. There is no part of the body, no organ of the body, no cell of the body, that is without its own mental being or nature.

When this important fact is understood and perceived, the fundamental explanation of mental healing is understood. The student no longer speaks of the power of "mind over matter," for he sees that it is really a manifestation of **mind over mind**. Of one kind of mind over another kind of mind. This fact being grasped thoroughly, the whole system of mental cure is perceived as a reasonable and logical idea, instead of a theory opposed to the accepted facts of Nature.

Just as the activities of the brain cells in performing their own assigned work are so closely correlated and combined that they are regarded as a unity, and form our thinking "mind" as a whole; so are the activities of our cells, parts, organs and other members of our bodies so closely correlated and combined in their actions and interaction that they form a unity, and may be regarded as one mind working in harmony and unity. For the want of a better name the combined mind many be called "The Corporeal Mind." This term will be used to indicate this great indwelling mind which is the active spirit of our physical functions and bodily life.

The Corporeal Mind must not be thought of as dwelling apart and separate from the other fields of mental activity. In fact, no part of this field of activity in the human being, whether physical or psychical, so dwells apart. Everything is correlated, interdependent, and interactive. All coordinated and harmonious parts of one whole.

The Corporeal Mind is really one of the phases or planes of that great field of human mentality known as the Subconscious Mind. The Subconscious Mind performs about 80% of the mental activity of the person. The remaining 20% being left for the Conscious Mind to perform. Just as the Conscious Mind consists and is composed of the many faculties of sensation, perception, thought, etc., so is the Subconscious Mind composed of numerous distinct planes or field of subconscious mental activity.

The Corporeal Mind, like all other phases or aspects of the Subconscious Mind, responds to the ideas, suggestions, and orders given to it by the Conscious Mind of its owner. And, it also accepts the ideas, suggestions, and commands of others unless its owner orders it not to. This important psychological fact explains the undoubted occurrence of causing disease by the accepted ideas and suggestions of others, or of one's own conscious mind. And, likewise, the cure and removal of disease by the same causes.

Before going into the details of The Corporeal Mind we should examine the fact of acceptance of the ideas and suggestions, or auto suggestions, by the Corporeal Mind, and its response to them.

There are several general laws which govern the activities of the Subconscious Mind. They manifest universally and may be always expected to exert their influence. These laws are as follows:

(1) The Subconscious Mind accepts as true any idea suggested to it, or impressed upon it; UNLESS (a) there already exists in the Subconscious Mind a contrary idea sufficiently strong enough to counteract the new one; OR (b) the Subconscious Mind has acquired a certain mental trend, or habit of thought, which is opposed to the introduction of the new idea; OR (c) the Subconscious Mind is **commanded** by its owner not to receive or accept such suggestions or ideas, or classes of ideas.

(2) The Subconscious Mind proceeds to logically manifest the conclusion of the suggested and accepted idea; to make it take form in action or physical condition; to adopt it as habit of manifestation and action.

(3) The Subconscious Mind will continue to manifest along the lines of the accepted suggested idea until either (a) it is neutralized, cancelled, and replaced by a sufficiently strong opposing idea or suggestion; OR (b) the accepted suggested idea is traced back to its birth in the mind of the person, and is shown to be erroneous, based on wrong premises, and therefore untrue; in both of which cases it is manifest, OR to be more exact, it is thus **painted over** by the new and true idea, and ceases to appear in the mind, or to manifest in action or form.

The student is cautioned against regarding the term "suggestion" to mean any mysterious use of the mind; or as being confined to certain forms of ideas. The term "suggestion" means merely an indirect idea, an argument or piece of advice. It is distinguished from argument, or logical proof, by the absence of formal evidence or discussion. A suggestion is usually an idea which seems plausible, and which is advanced with an air or appearance of truth, reality, or accepted fact. An "auto-suggestion" is a suggestion advanced from the conscious mind of the person himself, usually derived from the "working over" of ideas which he has heard but which were not accepted at the time. Although when the person is aquatinted with the psychology of suggestion he may deliberately form ideas which he deliberately "auto-suggests" to his Subconscious Mind as facts.

Ideas are suggested and accepted by the Subconscious Mind in a number of ways, of which the following are the most important:

1. **Authority.** Persons are strongly affected by ideas suggested with an air or appearance of authority. Persons exercising authority, such as priests and preachers, teachers and instructors, physicians, lawyers, judges, persons in charge of and directing other people, writers, public speakers, etc., manifest an appearance of authority, and speak in tones of authority, hence their suggestions carry with them a weight which in many cases is out of all proportion to their truth or real value.

2. **Obedience or Imitation.** Persons accept implicitly, in many cases, the ideas of those around them. They imitate the mental states of others and accept their ideas, and belief becomes of the influence in numbers. Example "everyone thinks so-and-so" takes the place of proof in their minds. More than this they "take on" the physical conditions of those around them for the same reason. The Subconscious Mind is quite imitative and readily falls into the habit of accepting the beliefs, ideas and conditions of those around its owner.

3. **Association.** Persons accept easily suggested ideas which resemble other ideas which they have previously accepted. They associate the new idea with the old one, although there may be little or no resemblance between them. Consequently, shrewd and unscrupulous men sometimes impose upon honest people in this way. Example: they make

themselves, or their proposition appear like some other person or proposition which has been satisfactory to the person, and this associated sameness disarms the person and causes him to accept the suggested idea far more readily than he would have otherwise. The confident man, charlatan, and faker operates along these lines of suggestion. And, likewise, many people accept suggestions concerning their physical condition because of this fancied resemblance to something else, which they otherwise would have refused to notice.

An important law of suggestion is this: **Suggestion gains force by repetition.** The first suggestion may make a little impression but the same suggestion repeated frequently makes a deeper and longer lasting impression with each repetition. Until finally the idea is firmly impressed upon the Subconscious Mind of the person.

We won't go into the important results of suggestion at this time; for we are concerned merely with those which produce physical effects for now. When the Subconscious Mind accepts suggested ideas relating to physical conditions, functioning, health, etc., it at once passes the idea over to the Corporeal Mind. The Corporeal Mind then proceeds to manifest into reality and physical form and function the idea given, which it accepts as truth in absence of opposing ideas.

In this way many people have developed conditions of disease from purely mental causes, and many have died from the logical development of such diseases. Many people are made ill from fear and suggestions of contagion and infection. Many people acquire disease by reason of vivid pictures placed in their minds through reading newspaper descriptions of disease, patent medicine advertisements, etc. It is a fact known to all officials of the medical schools that students frequently "take on" all the symptoms of the diseases they are studying about in their text books.

And, likewise, the law works with equal force in the opposite direction. For all the cures made by the faith healers, prayer curists, divine healers, and other practitioners of the same kind; and by the practitioners of Mental Healing, suggestive therapy, and similar scientific methods of applying the power of the mind to cure physical disease; are really based upon this fundamental principle. This may seem strange to the student when first stated but a careful examination of the facts of the case will bring to him such an overwhelming proof of its correctness, that it will seem strange to him that anyone can doubt it.

Remember, though, that Therapeutic Suggestion means **simply the indirect placing of an idea in the Subconscious Mind in such a way that it is accepted as truth, and therefor manifested in action, form, and functioning by that phase of the Subconscious Mind known as the Corporeal Mind, which has control of the functions and activities of the physical body.**

3 THE CELLS OF THE BODY

If you are studying physiology and psychology you cannot expect to have a sound base and foundation for this structure of knowledge unless you become thoroughly familiar with the nature and character of the cells of which the entire human body is composed.

The corporeal cells are those very minute elementary structures of which the organic tissues are composed. By tissues we mean the elementary materials, varying in structure and function, which compose the bodily organs, members, and parts. And, consequently, the cell is the physical base of the activity of the Corporeal Mind. So, from the position of both physiology and of psychology the cell is the logical subject of the beginning of study and investigation.

The corporeal cells are very minute; in fact they are microscopic. From them the muscles, tissues, nerves, blood, bones, hair and nails are built. From the hardest enamel of the tooth to the most delicate and soft tissue of the mucous membrane, the human body is found to be composed of cells. And these cells are, for all practical purposes of comparison, identical with the single cells which exist as independent entities or living creatures in the lowest form of the life scale. Every human body is in reality a great community of cells, grouped and associated, coordinated and combined for cooperative work and functioning, yet each is a separate living organism.

Each of these cells has a nucleus in the center which is the most vital part of its being. The nucleus of the cell is its central life force. Which may be compared to the yolk of an egg. It is more complex than the general substance of the cell, and seems to contain within itself the essence of the life and being of the cell. The cells reproduce themselves by growth and division; they are born, perform their tasks, give birth to others cells, and then die.

The cells preserve a certain degree of individuality and separateness, though their work is performed by reason of their tendency to combine with other cells into groups and these into still larger groups and so on. A constant relation being maintained between the members of each group and so on until all the cells in the body are considered as a great group connected in all of its parts and divisions.

Now, let's take a look at the work performed by these wonderful little bits of living substance, in their various groupings and associations with each other. Physiology recognizes about forty different kinds of cells, yet all belong to the one great family of cells. Their differences are merely adaptions to function, work and purpose.

For example: the muscle cells, which are adapted to their work of contracting the muscles which they compose. Then there are the connective tissue cells which join together and form the tough fibrous tissue which binds together and protects the various parts of the organism. Then again, we find the bone cells which select, arrange and set in place the lime material of which the bony parts of the body is composed. Then we find the several groups of cells which select and place in position the silicate mineral substances which are needed to form the nails, the hair, and other similar parts of the body. Then there are the gland cells which work industriously to secrete the fluids needed in digestion and similar vital processes. Then we discover the very active family of blood cells which members work to build up and repair the various parts of the system and do the scavenger work of carrying off the debris of the system to be burned up by the oxygen in the lungs. And, passing over many equally important families of cells, we finally come to the family of brain and nerve cells, where the work of rendering possible all feeling, thinking and acting of the human being is performed.

The cell families of the body are like a great cooperative community, each cell and each group of cells performing its own work in the community, each acting for its own good, and the good of its particular group, and at the same time for the good of the entire body of cells. You must remember that the body exists only as a body of cells. A great cooperative community of cells. It is not sufficient to say and think that "the body has cells" but rather "the body is a collection of cells" or even "the cells are formed into a body of cells."

Some of the cells are on the active line, while others are held in reserve to be called upon when needed. Some are stationary, while others remain stationary until called into motion. And a third general class is always moving about.

Some of the cells carry burdens of material from place to place, building material needed by certain stationary cells performing work. Other cells perform scavenger work and gather up the garbage of the system. Other cells perform police work and arrest intruders in the system, often times locking them up by building a wall around them. Other cells form the army which repels the microbes and germs of disease which have invaded the system. The cells of the nervous system form a living information wire, joining hands (so to speak) and passing along the messages from one end of the line to the other.

The number of cells in the human body is countless. A faint idea of their almost infinite number may be formed by considering the fact that in each cubic inch of blood there are over seventy five thousand millions of red blood cells alone, not taking into consideration the millions of other kinds of cells.

The red blood cells travel along in the blood flowing through the arteries and veins. Taking up a supply of oxygen from the lungs and carrying it through the arteries to the various parts of the body, where they deliver it to the cells requiring it for vital processes. Then, starting on their return journey through the system they gather up the waste products and this debris is finally consumed in the crematory of the lungs and thrown off as carbonic acid gas by breath. Some of these cells force their way through the wall of the arteries, veins and tissue when called upon for repair work.

Your body is constantly undergoing change; constantly breaking down cells and constantly repairing the damaged places with new cells. Our bodies, in all their parts, are being continuously made over. All of the work of this kind, whether it be the growth of new hair or finger nails, or the slower processes of other parts of the body, is performed by these minute workers, the cells.

Perhaps as typical, and as interesting as example of this work of the cells, is that of the healing of a wound. Let us consider this in order to have a clear idea of the work performed by cells. Here is the process:

First the body is discovered to be wounded by some outside force. The tissues, and often the glands, muscles and nerves are severed. The wound begins to bleed, and its sides separate. The nerves carry the message of trouble to the brain where a "call for help" is sent out. The cells rush to the area to begin the process of healing. The flowing blood washes away the dirt to prevent infection and then starts coagulating to form a protective substance that resembles glue and then afterward develops into a scab.

The repair cells arrive at the injury to start work of connecting the tissues by bringing together the sides of the wound, and knitting the tissue cells together. And here is manifested an almost unbelievable degree of "Mind." The cells of the tissues, blood vessels, etc., on both sides of the wound begin to reproduce themselves rapidly, each cell growing and separating itself into two, and these into two and so on until there is sufficient material created to do the repair work. These new cells increasing in number reach forward from each side of the wound until finally meeting and connecting with the cells on the other side. The connective tissues cells connect with the connective tissue cells on the other side; the blood vessel cells connect with their own kind on the other side; the nerve cells do the same until finally there is a complete bridge built, each various parts of each side being connected with the same kind of parts on the other side.

After this internal repair work is made, the skin cells start to work and build a new skin over the area. The whole process shows purposeful action, a coordinated effort and an undoubted presence of mental direction. It is useless for materialists to speak of mechanical and chemical laws as an explanation of such vital process as this. The most skeptical observer, if he is honest with himself, is forced to admit that there is manifested the activities of living, thinking, minute creatures, coordinated and regulated, directed and guided by some mental center higher than themselves. It is impossible to doubt this any more than one would doubt that the work of the bees in the hive is a vital manifestation. It is not enough to call it "instinctive" for instinct itself is a name given to only one phase of mental activity.

A clear understanding of the mental activities of cells will give us a key of understanding to the secret of mental healing.

4 MINDS OF THE CELLS

In the preceding lesson we have seen the wonderful work performed by the cells of which the human body is composed. Can there be any doubt that these cells are alive and have Mind within them? Any other assumption would be ridiculous. The single cells found in the lower stages of animal and vegetable life, which perform even less complicated and complex actions are regarded as living, thinking creatures. So there can be no reason for denying life and Mind to the cells which compose the human body and which constitute a great cooperative community.

Biology teaches us that every living thing is possessed of sufficient mind to enable it to perform its tasks and adjust to its environment. Even the tiny cells are possessed of sufficient mind to enable them to preserve their lives, perform their work, and reproduce their species. The cells in the human body have sufficient mind to enable them to seek, select, and absorb food, and to move from one place to another in search for it when necessary. They have mind enough to enable them to perform the complicated work referred to in the preceding lesson. The intelligence shown in the work of the red blood cells is brilliant and is an undoubted proof of the existence of a high degree of Mind in the cells. The other work performed by the other cells, such as the selection of mineral matter needed for building up bone, hair, and nails, is no less brilliant!

Eminent biologists have conducted careful research of the life activities of cells and have discovered some very important facts regarding them. It was discovered the cells manifest rudimentary memory which enables them to learn by experience and to avoid the recurrence of unpleasant happenings. They show their likes and dislikes very plainly and they exhibit the tendency to acquire habits. Some researchers insist that they even show evidence of purposeful preparation for future action and act in anticipation of the future.

But the mind in the cells is more than just the particular manifestation of mind in each particular cell. There is also found a sympathetic and coordinated mental activity existing between all the individual cells of the body. There are groups of cells existing in the body for each organ and part. Just how these cells coordinate and cooperate in this way is unknown to science, there seems to exist a high form of telepathic communication between them, of which we get a hint of in the psychology of human crowds. There is a "contagion of thought" between the various members.

The cells possess mind not only for their own purpose or task but also mind to combine and work for the purpose of the group of cells and also for the complete group composing the body. The combination of the cell groups into organ groups of cells is so complete and thorough that to all intents and purposes each organ of the body may be regarded as a living creature, having a mind of its own. This is no false imagination, but is a scientific fact of biological psychology. Each organ has its own mind and uses it in its own activities. When that mind becomes impressed upon with erroneous ideas it begins to manifest abnormally and when it is restored by properly directed mental treatment it resumes its normal functioning.

For those that think this collective mentality of the cells composing the body is unthinkable, we would suggest a study of the action of collective mentality in the various life forms. For instance, observation of a school of fish that seems to move by a common impulse, as if under the action of a collective mind. The same phenomenon being noted in the case of flocks of birds, herds of animals and even in crowds of people. The actions of bees in a hive show such a close coordination that the animating spirit moving them has been called "the spirit of the hive."

Students of human psychology have noted the characteristics of the psychology of human crowds, audiences, congressions, mobs, etc. It is a proven fact of psychology that the various individuals composing a crowd of people think, say and do things when in the crowd that would normally be foreign to them as separate individuals. There is a strange "contagion of thought" among the individuals of a crowd. Each individual in a crowd loses a certain degree of individuality and acquires a greater degree of collective mentality. He becomes a member or part of the "collective mind" of the crowd; at the same time the crowd itself takes on a being of its own, which disappears when the crowd is dissolved.

Observations prove that an individual immerged for a length of time in a crowd in action soon finds himself in a special state, which most resembles a state of fascination or hypnosis. The conscious personality has entirely vanished and will and discernment are lost. All feelings and thoughts are bent in the favor of the hypnotizer. An individual in a crowd is a grain of sand amid other grains of sand which the wind stirs up at will.

All of the above leads us to the inevitable conclusion that the same general principle of "collective mind" manifests in the case of the various organs and parts of the body. Every facet of physiology seems to sustain this idea and the idea itself is based upon the foundations of biology and psychology. The liver has its own collective mind as does the heart, stomach, kidneys, nervous system and so on. Each of these collective minds has its own unique characteristics and qualities. And, all combined in collective mental coordination, compose the entire body itself.

Individual cells are the units of which the whole body is built. Our Corporeal Mind is, in elemental form, cell mind. And so, at last, all disease must originate in the cells and all cures must be directed toward the cells. The cell minds of course being the soul and spirit of activity of the cell.

The best therapeutic theory today states that all disease is a failure of the cells to function properly, to do their own work, to repair and to eliminate waste matter. This improper functioning may be the fault of individual cells, or it may result from a failure of cell groups (large or small) to cooperate properly and to work in harmony. Sometimes there is manifested an actual rebellion of the cells or groups of cells. These failures of the cells to do their appointed work properly results in either local or general conditions of disease or ill health. Naturally, it follows that the diseased condition may be cured only by restoring the cell activities to natural function.

Nature often performs this curative work by bringing pressure to the mind in the cell or group of cells but sometimes the Mind itself becomes obsessed with the delusion of disease and in such cases it must be restored to normal conditions by treatment from the outside. Here is where Mental Healing performs its great work. By reaching the mind in the cells and in the cell groups the abnormal condition is neutralized and destroyed so the normal condition may be restored. Even in cases in which there exists a material or mechanical cause for the disorder, proper stimulation of the mind in the cells and organs sets up an increased resistive and combative power and the forces are rallied and directed toward the removal of the existing obstacle.

Mental Healing is not necessarily bound up with metaphysical, philosophical or theological theories. Instead, it is based on the combined discoveries of biology, physiology and comparative psychology. There is a biological and physiological basis of cure underlying the theory and practice of Mental Healing which is often lost sight of by the acceptance of metaphysical theories, philosophical hypotheses and theological dogmas which they have attached to the general subject of mental healing.

No matter how far away you seem to get in your studies, from the cell and its mind, the basis of the system is to be found in the presence of the mind in the cells of which the human body is composed.

5 THE SYMPATHETIC NERVOUS SYSTEM

Nature, or the Power that is behind Nature, has built up an intricate system of nerves, nerve centers and nerve connectors by means of which the Mind is able to perform the complex activities and functions of the body which is composed of cells and cell groups. The largest part of this work is performed by a part of the nervous system few people have ever heard of or have become familiar with.

We are in the habit of thinking of Cerebral Spinal Nervous System when we think of the "nervous system" so we ignore the existence of the Sympathetic Nervous System which performs all of the unconscious, involuntary activities of the body. Such as the actions of the heart, stomach, liver, kidneys, etc. and which also attends to the important processes of secretion, nutrition, excretion, reproduction, etc.

The term "sympathetic" was originally applied to this great system of nerves and nerve centers because there is a reciprocal action of the different cell groups and parts of the body, one with another, in apparent "sympathy" with each other. A disturbance in one part of the body sets up a disturbance of activity in other parts. The whole body suffers in sympathy with an injured or diseased part or member. Thus, a wound will produce fever, stomach trouble or indigestion, headaches, etc. The secretions of the body respond quickly in "sympathy" with the conditions in other parts of the body.

The Sympathetic Nervous System consists of a great cable of nerves running from the base of the scull to the coccyx or end of the spinal column, but not within the spinal column itself, as is the case with the cerebrospinal cable or spinal cord. These cables run on each side of the body by the side of the vertebrae and bunch out into ganglia or nerve centers along their course. These cables are connected by branch lines with spinal nerves and with other nerves of the cerebrospinal system and are also connected with the branches running to all of the organs of the body.

The Cerebrospinal Nervous System is concerned with our conscious activities and all of our conscious motions and work is performed by means of it. The Sympathetic Nervous System preforms the unconscious and involuntary motions and functions. By means of this latter system our hearts beat, our lungs inspire and expire, the blood circulates, the stomach and intestines perform their work of digestion and assimilation, the liver and kidneys and the glands of the body secrete the important juices, and the entire reparative and nutritive work of the body is performed. The Sympathetic Nervous System and the Mind that animates and directs its activities never sleep or rest. They are always at work while the Conscious Mind and its Cerebrospinal System rest in sleep about one third of the time.

An important feature of the Sympathetic Nervous System is its series of ganglia, or knots of gray nerve matter, which are scattered through the body, particularly along the side of the spine. Each ganglion is a complex center having branches radiating in several directions. In several places these ganglia are grouped together in still more complex arrangement, called a plexus (plural "plexi"). The principal plexus is the well-known "Solar Plexus" which some have called the "Abdominal Brain" by reason of its high power and complex arrangement. This important plexus is situated in the upper part of the abdomen almost directly back of the "pit of the stomach" it is the center from which emerge nerves extending in all directions. This great center is regarded as the Central Office or headquarters of the Mind.

The Mind is really the animating spirit of the sympathetic nervous system and the organs controlled by it. Consequently, you will find that whatever affects the Mind must reflect through the sympathetic nerves upon the entire body controlled by its power. The way to reach the organs is through the Mind by means of its great chain of sympathetic nerves. This is the scientific explanation of the process of mental healing.

In the case of the reparative work of the cells performed after a wound has been caused to the body, it is the Mind that directs and guides the energies of the cells via the orders being transmitted over the wires of the sympathetic nervous system. A general alarm is sent out and all cells are called into service. And, as in the case of all natural healing, this is often called natures healing force. For the Mind is not only the great regulator and governor of the physical activities, but also the great natural physician of the body.

As an instance of the control of the Mind over the body, we have an excellent example in the regulation of the circulation of the blood. The blood does not flow through the body in a regular, invariable manner, in response to purely mechanical laws as so many believe. On the contrary, the Mind regulates the flow in accordance with the circumstances of the moment. When necessary millions of tiny capillaries are closed or opened up in order to increase or decrease the blood supply to certain parts. The blood supply of each organ is regulated by the needs of that organ at that time, as determined by the Mind governing it. Even the rate of the pulsations of the heart is under the control of the Mind and varies according to circumstances.

The healing of a wound; the knitting together of a broken bone; the complex arrangements made necessary by the processes of gestation and child birth and thousands of other manifestations of unconscious mind in physical processes; all these are the work of the Mind working with its sympathetic nervous system. When we speak of "Nature" doing this or that in the work of helping along the curative work or vital processes of the body we are referring to this

Mind acting through its sympathetic nervous system.

The Mind is animated by two very important motives: (1) the motive of self-preservation and (2) the motive of the reproduction of the species. All of its work is along these two lines. These are the only two laws of action that it recognizes. This is why it strives to preserve health in the body and also why it exerts a sometimes overpowering influence in the matter of sexual attraction.

Much of what we call sickness is really the effect of the Mind to throw out of the system morbid and injurious material which has gathered there. Fever is often the attempt of the Mind to burn up this debris which it fails to get rid of otherwise. If it is unable to get rid of the cause of the trouble, it tries to adjust itself to the impaired conditions and strives to balance the physical functions so as to get the best possible results under the unfavorable conditions. The Mind is ever working toward life and health for its owner. Sometimes it undertakes heroic and even desperate methods in order to combat and defeat particularly dangerous conditions.

A careful investigation shows that the "Nature" of medical science is really mental in its nature and is identical with our conception of the Mind. Mind is ever at work in the physical processes of nutrition, elimination, reproduction and the reparative processes of cure. The basis of all true healing is to be found in this Mind.

The Subconscious Mind sometimes lags in its work or becomes sluggish and apathetic or perhaps discouraged from some cause or another. In such cases it may be stimulated to action and even guided and set to work in the proper direction by means of incentive coming through the Conscious Mind or directed immediately to itself. This fact makes possible all forms of mental healing no matter what name they may operate under or what theory they may proceed; the basic fact remains the same.

The rule works both ways! For we find that much disease is caused, maintained and perpetuated by means of wrongful suggestions or ideas implanted in the Mind by means of influence, suggestion, teaching, advice or other methods of implanting an idea into the mind. The Mind, though very set in its way as a rule, is affected by suggestion or wrong ideas if strongly and repeatedly presented to it. And when it finally is affected by these ideas, it manifests its false belief by means of its very efficient system of sympathetic nerves reaching to all parts of the body where disease and improper functioning begins. Next to false ideas, fear is the most potent factor in this mental causation of disease. Fear paralyzes the activities of the Mind and prevents it from doing its work properly and efficiently.

It is hoped that you will not pass over these basic and fundamental explanations on the ground they are "dry reading." Such a course would be very foolish for it is necessary that these fundamental and basic principles of the theory of the cause and cure of disease be thoroughly grasped and remembered in order that the principals of healing may have an intelligent foundation.

6 MENTAL CAUSES OF DISEASE

A mind turned in the wrong direction will surely cause disease as a mind turned in the right direction will cure disease. The mental motive power runs when reversed and well as when turned forward.

Medical science, in its history, has taken note of many instances of great mental epidemics, accompanied by physical illness, disease and death. Fear is contagious, as all physicians know, and when it is based on a strong belief in a suggested idea of disease, the disease spreads rapidity. The pages of the records of medical science are filled with the testimony of physicians regarding this evil potency of mind in the direction of causing disease.

The records of physiological psychology contain many references to cases in which serious illness and even death have been caused by the efforts of practical jokers to "scare" their victims. The usual plan is to have several persons during the course of a few hours tell the victim that he is looking very ill and that his appearance resembles that of another friend who grew suddenly ill and then died. The usual result is that the victim will become frightened and in some cases will be actually prostrated with weakness and compelled to take to his bed.

Medical students frequently contract the diseases whose symptoms they have been studying in their text books. Specialists in medical practice frequently contract the very disease that they have been studying and treating in their practice. The strong mental image tends to influence the Mind and that manifests in physical disorder. Many people have contracted diseases described in detail in the patent medical records and other fear producing printed matter describing the disease for which the medicine is intended.

Medical records also contain numerous references to cases in which people have died from the belief and fright arising from having taken what they have supposed to be poison, but which in reality was some harmless drug. Cases are known in which patients died after having manifested all the symptoms of poisoning by the drug that they had supposed they had taken, but of which an autopsy failed to reveal even a trace.

The well authenticated instances of the production of stigmata, or the marks of the nails on the hands and feet of the crucified Savior, on the bodies of religious devotees who have too long contemplated the crucifix, is an instance of the power of the Mind over the body which it controls. Suggestionists have produced blisters and even scars on the arms of patients, by suggesting that the harmless court plaster placed on the arm was a strong irritant chemical. Strong sympathy, accompanied by a vivid imagination, has caused people to suffer the pain being undergone by others. In many cases even faint pink marks corresponding to the scars on the injured person have appeared on the body of the sympathetic relative or friend. It is a fact of common experience that many men suffer from the sympathetic nausea during the pregnancy of their wives and as many more experience soreness and pain around the lower part of the spine accompanying the labor pains of their wives during the birth of their children.

Hair has turned grey from emotion, milk has been rendered poisonous in the breasts of nursing mothers, from similar causes, it is frequent that nausea is produced by some story relating to disgusting details, or even from the memory of a similar occasion, the thought of certain acid fruits, a lemon for instance, will cause the water to flow from the mouth, the bowels are frequently moved after one has thought of some unpleasant cathartic medicine one has taken in the past, physicians know that menstruation in one woman frequently results in a similar happening in the case of other women around the first one who became aware of the fact, even though their regular monthly periods have not as yet arrived.

Example of the case in which a lady saw three fingers cut from the hand of a child in an accident. She was so affected that her hand began to pain her and swelling resulted. The three fingers on her hand corresponding to those cut from the hand of the child became so badly inflamed an incision became necessary to evacuate the puss that had formed.

The unconscious mind as revealed that hypnosis can exercise marvelous control over the nervous, vaso-motor, circulatory and other systems. There seems to be no reasonable grounds for doubting that, in certain chosen subjects, congestion, burns, blisters, bleeding from the nose or skin can be produced by suggestion. The significance of this lies in the fact that the hypnotic state is now recognized as one in which suggestion has an exaggerated effect. Suggestion in the waking state or even the auto suggestion of the person himself, operates along the same lines and sometimes in quite a marked degree.

As for the effect of "pure imagination" on the body, under the suggestion and belief in placebos or other "make believe" remedies every physician can supply numerous evidences. Some physicians with a greater scientific curiosity than a regard for their patients have produced almost at will the entire range of physical conditions by prescribing harmless and inactive chemical substances accompanied with the strong suggestion of their effect. And as every physician knows only too well a hysterical patient will manage to counterfeit and thus eventually to actually induce a great range of physical disorders.

We could fill an entire book on instances of this kind. The one principle which is illustrated in all of these cases is this: That the Mind which has control of the functions of the physical body, from great to small, simple to complex, is amenable to suggestion or insinuated ideas. Either those suggestions of other people or those which are "picked up" by the conscious mind of the person himself. The suggestions or insinuated ideas, once accepted, tend to manifest in action and outward expression and thus cause to appear in physical form and conditions that which originally existed in the mind alone.

From this it is seen that the real cause of many cases and forms of physical disorders and disease is to be found in these suggested or acquired ideas or thoughts which have been accepted by the Mind and subsequently manifested into objective forms, states and conditions.

Consequently, the practitioner of Mental Healing must always look for these mental causes of the diseases which he is called upon to treat and heal. While, of course, he must direct his treatment to the physical conditions as they exist at the time strive to reach and remove the original erroneous idea or thought which has really caused the whole trouble. In this way he discovers and removes the roots of the trouble and does not limit himself with merely treating and removing the symptoms.

In chapter 2 (lesson 2) we have seen that the Subconscious Mind (of which the Mind is a phase or aspect of) will continue to harbor and manifest these erroneous ideas and thoughts until the following things happen: (a) the idea is neutralized, cancelled and replaced by a sufficiently strong opposing idea or suggestion or (b) the accepted suggested idea is traced back to its birth in the mind of the person and is shown to be erroneous based on wrong premises and untrue. In both of these methods the erroneous and harmful idea is wiped from the tablets of the mind and ceases to exist or express it otherwise. The erroneous idea is painted over by the new and true idea and ceases to appear in the mind or to manifest in form and action.

This point of practice is worthy of special emphasis and of careful thought and remembrance for it goes right to the root of the problem and eradicates the seed of the foul growth that is causing the trouble. Too often the mental healer, like the medical doctor, contends himself with treating and removing the outward symptoms of the internal problem. Try to discover the root of the trouble and manage to kill it at the same time you are healing the manifestations arising from its presence in the mind of the patient. This and this alone is true and complete mental healing of the disease.

7 THE PRINCIPALES OF CURE

It is a fundamental principle of Mental Healing that all forms of cures of diseases are really but different phases of mental cure. In all healing processes the active principle is always found to be the mind in the cells, cell groups, organs, or in the body as a whole. The healing power of Nature performs the curative work of the body and is mental in its elemental nature; therefore, all cures are mind cures.

The healing processes of the body are not blind forces or mechanical energies; they are characteristically mental in their activities. There is intelligence at work in these processes, instinctive and subconscious; it still manifests all the characteristics of intelligence. There is always manifesting of a working plan and purpose, and an endeavor of the Mind to accomplish the results indicated in the plan and purpose.

When we consider that each cell and each group of cells is a living, mental something and not mechanical, inert, lifeless thing moved only by external forces, the energies of the cell abide within the cell and manifest in accordance with intelligent processes. The curative process always consists of the repairing of waste tissues and creating a harmonious readjustment of mental relations and conditions by the activities of the cells.

Even when external remedies and methods are used they are seen to be merely the supplying of the cells with proper stimuli, nourishment and aid. Or the removal of those mechanical or other obstacles from their way. The Mind in the body, organs and cells performs all the real curative work. All else is but an aid or help to the mental force within the body, organ or cells.

The physician may remove undesirable and harmful substances from the system making it easier for the cells to perform the task of the Mind within the body. Or the surgeon may clean and drain the wound, thus taking a portion of the work from the cells and rendering it easier for them to do their work. Or the surgeon may place the broken bones and hold them back together with bandages allowing then the Mind in the cells to do their healing work and knit them together. **Man aids, but Nature heals.**

More than this, medical science recognizes the fact that disease is not a foreign something that attacks the system. What is called "disease" is in many cases the symptoms of the efforts of Nature to eliminate objectionable and harmful conditions and to resume normal states of functioning and activity. The theory of many thoughtful physicians is that disease is frequently really a self-preservation action on the part of Nature. An action by which she seeks to preserve the body by setting up conditions which have arisen. If Nature is unable to throw off the abnormal conditions, it at least accommodates itself to the new state of affairs and strives to make the best of it. To manage to get the best possible results or the least possible measure of harm.

There is no denying that anything that will aid the mental action of the cells, organs and body in its reparative work must aid the cure. And here is where Mental Healing comes in. Nothing can aid and strengthen, direct and sustain the mind in the cells, organs and body better than the Mind itself. Whatever strengthens the Mind and directs its energies effectively must materially aid in the work of the cure. And this is what is accomplished with Mental Healing. The Mind under the proper stimulus will not only manifest latent powers and energies but it also obey the direction and guidance of a phase of mind more positive than itself and act more efficiently. Upon this fundamental principle of practice all scientific mental healing is based.

When this principal of healing – the principal that all cures are really performed through cell activity and that the cell activity is mental and under the control of the confederated minds of the total cell life of the body – is clearly perceived, then the mystery of Mental Healing vanishes. For when this principal is grasped you will understand that all cures are really mental cures, no matter by what means or methods the mental forces are called into action. With this understanding it is seen that Mental Healing is simply the calling into action the mental forces resident in the cells, organs and entire physical system. Not by means of physical remedies or appliances but rather by a direct appeal to the Mind itself and to the cell minds and organ minds.

Mental healing. In any of its forms and phases, is the most direct and immediate form of healing there is. Instead of proceeding in a roundabout way to get at the mind in the cells, organs and parts to rouse it into activity it makes a direct appeal to the Mind and energizes it into activity. The Mind which is very amenable to suggestion or instructions properly given, agrees with the methods of cure stated to it by the healer or the person himself. It sends directing messages to the diseased organs and cells and stimulates them to greater activity producing harmony where discord has been manifested. It regulates and adjusts, directs and guides the activities of the cells and organs.

Although mental healing has been practiced from the beginning of time, under various names, forms and disguises and based upon many theories of varying degree of rationality the underlying principal has remained the same. The effect of all these varying methods and forms of treatment, plainly stated or else disguised under some fanciful theological or metaphysical theory, is identically the same. The rousing into activity and operation of the mind in the cells and organs of the body with the coordinated influence of the Mind. The cures are not made by reason of the theories, but in spite of them!

8 THE HISTORY OF MENTAL HEALING

The earliest forms of mental healing were those connected with the magicians, medicine men or primitive priests. From the beginning of time mankind has taken unto itself priests, magicians and medicine men. And, just as naturally as the proverbial duck takes to water, so have these priests, magicians and medicine men taken to the healing of disease. This is because the savage usually regards disease as something caused by the influence of devils and evil influences which must be chased away by the power of the magician or priest.

We, who can afford to smile at the superstition of these savages, must not make the mistake of supposing that these priests and magicians performed no cures. On the contrary, they did perform cures and their prototypes among the savage tribes of this day are still performing cures in the same way for the same reason.

The magic performances of these medicine men or magicians are directed toward the chasing away of demons of disease. They believe in the power of the demons and they believe in the power of the magicians... or else they wouldn't advertise their services. The attention and the imagination of the sick person are called into operation by the magic ceremonies. All students of Mental Healing understand the potency of the aroused imagination and expectant attention of a patient. This mental attitude results in a very curative and reparative activity on the part of the mind in cells and organs. The savage has a great amount of vital power, or vital mind, due to his natural ways of living and once this is directed toward the process, the cure begins to show marked improvement. The patient, noting the improvement, is encouraged in his faith and belief causing the reparative force of Nature to gain power until the cure is made.

The next form of healing we are going to look is that by religious ceremonies performed by priests. The priests claiming to be chosen instruments of the Deity, the natural claimed divine power of healing among other gifts. Their favorite method is "laying on of hands" accompanied by certain ceremonies of their particular religion. The literature and monumental remains of ancient Egypt, Greece, Rome, Persia, India and China show that the "laying on of hands" was a favorite and common method of cure in those days. There are evidences of it having been practiced nearly thirty-five hundred years ago in Egypt. It was also practiced extensively in ancient China and Persia several thousand years ago.

But this custom, so well established in the race, did not perish with the ancient religions. It has always been a feature of the Christian religion; in fact it formed one of the strong foundation stones of that religion in its early days. Healing the sick and casting out demons were two of the special offices of the early disciples and the priesthood naturally took over the privilege and practice when they replaced the early disciples.

In the Middle Ages healing by means of religious ceremonies, charms and blessings was very common. Sacred relics, alters, shrines and holy places were visited by great multitudes of people, many of whom experienced cures of their physical ailments. This practice has endured into this day in many parts of Europe. All over Europe you will find holy wells and holy shrines where miracles of healing are performed. The many crutches and other tokens of former illness which may be left at these holy places as a symbol of cure establish the fact the power has not departed from them. The power of the Mind aroused by faith and expectant attention still operates in the direction of the cure.

Later on some of the Kings and Queens took over the gift of healing, probably to the disgust of the priests whose revenues were affected. We find many records of "the Kings Touch" or "the Royal Touch" in the Middle Ages and beyond. There began a belief that touch of the hand of the monarch was a sure cure for disorders of the blood and skin. So at certain times of the year great multitudes would present themselves to the ruling monarch in order that they might be healed by his healing touch.

Those who may be inclined to smile at the idea of the monarch having and special power to heal should study the records of the times. Thousands were healed in this way without the assistance of medicine or surgery.

The great successes of Frauz Anton Mesmer in the later part of the eighteenth century are now perceived to have arisen by reason of the power of faith and expectant attention and not by any virtues of his theories of methods. He was followed by many who improved on his methods and built upon his theories. Braid, an English physician, 1841, dispelled the mystery of Mesmer's cures by advancing a new theory – that of Hypnotism. For a time many physicians followed Braid's methods and obtained great results. Then after that came the school of the French hypnotists, who evolved the theory of "Suggestion," which asserted that the healing power arose not from the hypnotic methods, but rather from the "suggestion" or mental commands given in the hypnotic state. Then others came along who discovered that Suggestion was equally effective when administered without any resort to hypnotism. This was the dawn of the modern scientific study of mental healing, for it revealed the important fact that in mental states, particularly those of faith and expectant attention, there was to be found a great healing power.

The great modern interest in, and improvement in the different methods of mental healing have arisen from the work of the practitioners of some of the many forms of "psychological healing," or "biological healing," all of which were offshoots of Mesmerism or Braidism. Gradually there sprung from this main trunk the several forms of Metaphysical Healing which became so popular and has grown remarkably.

The connecting link between the older schools of psychological healing, and the newer schools of metaphysical healing, is found in Dr. Phineas Parkhurst Quimby, a poor clock maker of limited education, but of a quick mind and a strong personality, who lived in Maine, one of the New England States of America. Quimby was attracted to the teachings of Mesmerism about 1838, and soon developed into a successful mesmeric healer. He followed along the lines of John Bovee Dod's "Electro-Biology" for a time, but soon evolved a more metaphysical theory of his own. His new conception was that disease arose from erroneous thinking, and that cures may be performed by getting the patient to think rightly. Among his pupils were Dr. Warren F. Evans and Julius A. Dresser, both of whom afterward established what they called "The Mind Cure," which was the direct ancestor of the great "New Thought" movement that was popular in America and Europe. Another patient and pupil of Dr. Quimby's was Mary Baker Eddy, who afterward founded the great Christian Science movement. Christian Science, however, now rejects the fact they all descend from Quimby.

Springing up as a result of the success of the Mental Science, Christian Science, and New Thought movements we find many instances of the desire of the people for religious and similar phases of mental healing. Divine healers by the score have appeared, flourished, and then disappeared. Francis Schlatter, the German shoemaker of Denver, Colorado, U. S. A., healed thousands of people who flocked to his cottage, believing him to be a prophet of God. John Alexander Dowie, an English preacher, created great interest, first in Australia and then in Chicago, Illinois, U. S. by his many cures. He established a church in Chicago, the walls of which were lined with crutches, trusses, etc., of persons who had been healed by his prayers and laying on of hands. Both Schlatter and Dowie have had many imitators, many of whom have met with more or less success.

The great New Thought movement, with its many divisions, and subdivisions, has a large following, and also has a great multitude of healers, all of whom make cures by the general methods of mental healing, though under many different theories and conceptions, and by many methods of application. Christian Science supports many fine churches and many healers and teachers, some of whom have grown wealthy as the result of their practice. The "Emmanuel Movement," started by some of the orthodox churches several years ago, is another illustration of the popularity of mental methods of healing and also of the common desire of the public to have such healing given under the cover, and in the form of religious teachings.

But don't imagine for a moment that any of the modern schools and phases of mental healing admit the true basis and foundation of their cures. On the contrary, they generally vigorously insist that their cures are made by reason of the truth of their particular theories and beliefs, or methods of treatment. They prefer the mystery and the possible monopoly of their own teachings.

But the cold-blooded scientific observer insists upon the fact of the simple, natural scientific basis and foundation, which always exists under the fanciful guises and forms. He sees that while each of the cults or schools has its own particular theory and teaching-each claiming that the other are lacking in truth; still each and every one of them are making cures, and in about the same proportion and percentage. Therefore, he claims that the truth lies not in any of their particular conceptions, but rather in a fundamental principle underlying them all, and common to all of their methods. This fundamental principle is that which forms the basis of these lessons; it is over and above any cult or school-it is based upon scientific observation and logical thought, and not upon revelation, inspiration; or religious dogma, or upon metaphysical innuendo.

9 MENTAL HEALING IN DISGUISE

As you may have already surmised, there are many cures created by the underlying principal of Mental Healing, which are not attributed to but which are giving credit to some other form of healing agency or power, method or principle.

Mental healing is the fundamental principle of mental cures. It being seen that all healing is really performed by the mind in the cells, organs and parts of the body and that this mind is under control of the Corporeal Mind and that the Corporal Mind takes up, accepts and acts upon the suggestions reaching it from the minds of others. Then it follows that mental cures may be made by agencies and methods which are accepted as efficacious by the Corporal Mind or rather by the subconscious mentality of which the Corporal Mind is a phase or part of.

In accordance with this principle of operation cures have been created by the most ridiculous and absurd methods and agencies, providing that the method of the agency was accepted as effective by the subconscious mind of the person. The belief in and faith in almost anything will act as a curative force along the lines as indicated. With this being said, we naturally look for the striking instances and examples of this natural law. The history of medicine is filled with instances and examples of this kind, many of which are very amusing when one views them in the light of the scientific principle involved.

It has been known to physicians for many centuries that the "imagination" of the patient, if sufficiently aroused, is capable of working many important cures. Physicians for centuries have laughed over this well-known fact.

It has long been the practice of physicians to administer "placebos" or make believe medicine in their practice when in doubt of the proper thing to prescribe. Colored water, strong flavored drops, pills and similar placebos have had their place in the list of remedies of most physicians. Originally intended to quiet the mind of the patient and to satisfy the demands of the friends and family of the sick person. Because of this these placebos have justified their existence and use. Physicians discovered that these placebos actually cause improvement and cures in many cases. The experience of any physician (if he is willing to admit it) will more than justify what we have just stated about placebos.

Depending on the belief of the patient a placebo could have therapeutic action. Many practitioners have stated that many of the drugs on their list have no other use than as a placebo. Some practitioners have obtained wonderful results from the use of placebos by assuring the patient that the drug will work. As long as the practitioner has belief and is able to impress it upon the patient. Other physicians, lacking in faith, fail to impress it upon the patient and have a less satisfactory result. An understanding of this principle has solved many mysteries of this kind.

Many cases of malaria were cured by giving the patient a charm with the word Febrifuge written on it. Fever and malaria and similar complaints have been successfully treated by common people using some sort of "pow wow" or mock "magic" treatment in which both the healer and the patient firmly believed. Seasickness and car sickness has also been cured with the use of placebos.

A woman in a London hospital was suffering from incurable paralysis of the spine for two years. She had spent all her money in treatments with no results and was brought to the hospital pending her admission to a rehabilitation facility. She was cured in two hours with the use of a placebo. Many cases of miracle cures such as this have been reported over the years.

The cures by use of herbal remedies can be accounted for in this same way. Same true for the "magnetic rings and bracelets" worn by some and also the other healing charms people carry. We see the advertisements and hear how they work "all cures" and even hear the testimonials from grateful patients. Our subconscious mind is listening to this information even if we are not consciously aware of it.

The student and practitioner of Mental Healing should become familiar with this class of mental cures – cases in which the cure is attributed to some material remedy, appliance or method, although really resulting from the mental principle called into operation. Once this is thoroughly understood, you then have the key to a whole new class of strange cures. This knowledge also prevents one from being led into error and being persuaded to "follow after strange gods" in healing. It also keeps you from being taken advantage of. Using this course of action on others is not recommended as a regular thing but there are cases in which the healer must take the material and work it into the proper shape by methods along the lines of least mental resistance. But you must never lose the true principle involved in the cure.

10 THREE METHODS OF MENTAL HEALING

While there are countless methods and processes of manifesting mental healing under the general principals of Mental Healing these methods may be grouped into three general principles of application. The student who thoroughly acquaints himself with the underlying principle of these three general classes will be master of the entire system. For all methods or forms of application are found to be some variation of one of these three or a combination of one or more of them.

Three general classes of methods for applying Mental Healing are as follows:

(1) Healing by Mental Suggestion
(2) Healing by Present Thought Induction
(3) Healing by Distant Thought Induction

The student should always remember that it is a very rare occurrence for any one of the above stated general methods to be used exclusively. In most cases there is always a greater result when you combine two or more of these methods.

For instance, the practitioner using Mental Suggestion almost always uses Personal Thought Induction in the presence of the patient, and often Distant Thought Induction when thinking of "the case" between treatments. In the same way, the practitioner using Direct Thought Induction always uses more or less Mental Suggestion (although they may do this unconsciously) when talking to the patient. He also uses Distant Thought Induction when thinking of "the case" between treatments. And the practitioner using Distant Thought Induction almost always uses Mental Suggestion when talking to the patient regarding treatment, and at the same time uses Personal Thought Induction when in the presence of the patient.

All of these methods facilitate cures by the same fundamental principle – that of stimulating into renewed and normal activity and functioning of the mind in the cells, organs and other parts of the body in the patient. The question of just what particular method to use is one of merely academic interest to the practitioner and the question of "how" to reach the mind of the affected parts.

You will soon discover that some forms of treatment are best adapted to the requirements of the patient. By understanding the fundamental sameness of the different methods and by acquainting yourself with the best ways of applying each one you will be equipped to handle effectively any kind of case that presents itself for treatment and to adapt this treatment to meet the needs of each patient.

The practitioner who allows himself to fall into the error of believing that only one method of mental healing is the "whole thing" and the only thing is placed at a disadvantage for obvious reasons. The wise practitioner is able to apply all the methods of mental healing in a scientific manner, rather than using narrow loyalty to a specific school or teacher. The best practitioner is one who "takes his own wherever he finds it" and applies it to his work. The true "eclectic" is one who takes what is best in many systems, and who wisely selects and boldly uses all methods of healing. There is no place for narrowness and one sidedness in Mental Healing if one wishes to become and remain a successful practitioner.

The three general classes of Mental Healing are as follows; when we consider each in its proper place we should consider the fundamental features and characteristics of each so that we may form a clear mental conception of each and perceive its place in the general system and principle of Mental healing.

(1) **Mental Suggestion**. Mental Suggestion is not hypnotic suggestion although in the public mind the two are usually regarded as the same. Hypnotic Suggestion is merely Mental Suggestion administered when the patient or subject is in the hypnotic state. The hypnotic condition is a state in which the Mental Suggestion has an exaggerated effect but it should be understood that the Mental Suggestion does not depend upon the presence of the hypnotic state. The best practitioners of Mental Suggestion do not seek to induce the hypnotic condition in their patients and in most cases they frown upon the practice of doing so.

The principle of Mental Suggestion is simply placing in the subconscious mind of the patient a firm, strong, positive idea of the physical condition sought to be induced in him. Suggestion differs from logical argument or reasoning and it does not seek to convince by logical proof but rather depends upon its acceptance by reason of its strong insistence and authoritative form of presentation. The principle underlying Suggestion is indicated by the original meaning of the Latin terms from which it derived, "suggero" meaning "to carry or place under." The technical meaning of "to suggest" is "to identify or introduce into the mind."

Suggestion: a process of communication of an idea to the subconscious mind in an unobtrusive manner, carrying conviction; when consciously there is no inclination for its acceptance and logically there are no adequate grounds for its acceptance. **"Suggestion enters into the understanding by the back stairs, while logical persuasion knocks at the front door."** Mental Suggestion in Mental Healing conveys to the mind of the patient the idea or mental picture of the physical condition sought to be induced and it conveys this by words, spoken, written or printed. The subconscious mind accepting the idea or picture so introduced passes it on the phase of itself known to us as the Corporal Mind and this in turn passes it on to the organ and cell minds concerned with that portion of the body in which the physical condition is sought to be induced or created.

This is one point to be remembered: **Mental Suggestion creates the desired idea in the Mind by means of words – spoken, written or printed.**

(2) **Personal Thought Induction**. By Personal Thought Induction the idea of the physical condition sought to be induced is introduced into the subconscious mind, and thus the Corporeal Mind, and to the cells and organs governed. This suggestion is not introduced by words as in the case of Mental Suggestion. There is a distinction here that you should remember.

Personal Thought Induction is always manifested when the practitioner is in the immediate personal presence of the patient. It is a known fact to students of advanced psychology that Thought, like magnetism or electricity, radiates from the thinker and coming in contact with the mental aura of the patient, tends to induce a corresponding idea, thought or mental picture of the physical condition which is sought to be induced in the patient.

These thought vibrations are not consciously perceived by the patient, instead they are taken up only by his subconscious mind and then passed on to the Corporeal Mind and then on to the cell and organ minds in his body. Once reaching the subconscious mind the process is identical with the process manifested in cases of Mental Suggestion. So you see the practical distinction between the two methods of Mental Healing so far considered. Mental Suggestion and Personal Thought Induction are simply the difference in reaching the subconscious mind of the patient. From that point the two processes are practically identical.

(3) **Distant Thought Induction**. In Distant Thought Induction we have the principle of Thought Induction plus the manifestation of certain mental powers which serve to carry the thought vibrations beyond the ordinary limits and range of Thought Induction. In this form of Thought Induction the principle of Thought Radiation is extended to become available even though many miles separate the practitioner from the patient.

In Distance Thought Induction the practitioner (a) creates in himself the mental idea and picture of the physical condition sought to be induced in the patient; same as Personal Thought Induction. And then (b) puts into operation certain powers of the mind and will, which serve to carry his thought vibrations to a distance. To project them into space to reach the distant patient, then (c) the vibrations reaching the subconscious mind of the patient are taken up, translated into ideas and pictures that correspond to those of the practitioner. These vibrations are then passed on to the Corporal Mind and into the cell minds and organ minds.

Now that you can see and understand the underlying principle of each and every one of these methods of manifesting Mental Healing is the same. They all reach the cell minds and organ minds of the patient through the subconscious mind and the Corporeal Mind of the patient. And by producing or inducing in these mental planes of the patient the idea and mental picture of the physical conditions sought to be created, produced or induced in him. This is the underlying principle of mental healing. The rest is a matter of application, technique and good judgement in selecting the best methods for each particular case.

11 MENTAL SUGGESTIONS

The principal of Mental Suggestion is based upon the fundamental fact that the mind of all human beings manifests a far greater range of activities on the subconscious level than on the conscious level. That nearly eighty percent of its activities are on the subconscious plane and that the subconscious level of the human mind is highly receptive and amenable to Suggestion.

Mental Suggestion does not depend upon logical processes or argumentative proof for its efficacy but bases its force and efficacy upon its positive appeal to the subconscious mind. The subconscious mind is by nature very receptive to suggestion and will instinctively accept any suggestion to it unless the conscious mind has forbidden the acceptance of the suggestion.

If the conscious mind is in a relaxed state, comfortable with its surroundings and trusting of the people around it (example: home environment or sacred space) then there is nothing to interfere with the acceptance of a suggestion by the subconscious mind, providing that the suggestions already accepted by it do not prevent the introduction of new and opposing ones. And, even in the last mentioned event, the old accepted suggestions may be neutralized by a constant flow of new suggestions of an opposite nature. This process has been compared to the flowing of clear water into a bowl of dirty water, in which case the overflow gradually carries off the diluted dirty water until the bowl is filled with perfectly clear water. This is what happens in most cases of Mental Healing by Mental Suggestion. The old negative suggestions are first diluted and then carried off being replaced by the new and positive ones.

The words of Mental Suggestion have no magic power in themselves; they represent ideas, which ideas are called into the mind by hearing or reading words. Sometimes colors and images are also attached to the ideas. Another point to remember is that Mental Suggestion is effective in proportion to the degree of feeling it arouses in the person to whom it is addressed. The reason of this last mentioned fact is that feeling always energizes an idea in the mind and makes it active and operative. The suggested idea or mental picture of a physical condition greatly desired by the patient is many times more active and effective than a suggested idea or mental picture of a condition which fails to arouse such feeling or desire.

Suggestions contain ideas and ideas are symbols of something thought or felt. The majority of ideas held in the mind of the race arise from feeling. People may not understand things but they have experienced feelings or emotions regarding them and have consequently formed many ideas from them. They do not always know the reason why an idea is held by them; they only know that they feel it that way. The majority of people are swayed and moved and act by reasons of induced feelings rather than the result of reasoning. When suggestion acts through the association of ideas, it is based upon the acquired impressions of the race, by which certain words, actions, manners, tones and appearances are associated with certain previously experienced feelings. It is true that suggestions may accompany an appeal to the reason or judgement of the person influenced and is generally used. But they constitute and appeal to a part of the mind entirely removed from reasoning and judgment. They are emotional first, last and all the time. Many personal appeals which are apparently made to reason are really made to the emotional side. One may subtly insinuate into an argument or conversation an appeal to the feelings or emotions of the hearer by an idea indirectly conveyed. Such an idea will be "felt" by the listener who will accept it into his own mind and before long he will regard it as one of his own thoughts. He will think that he thought it, when really he simply feels it and the feelings are induced.

Truth is merely words that are boldly asserted and plausibly maintained. The experienced practitioner of Mental Suggestion will at once recognize how appropriate that statement is when applied to the principle of suggestion. You will also recognize the fact that the power of a suggestion depends on the boldness, confidence and air of authority with which it is expressed. The effect of the suggestion will be greatly heightened by the introduction of some plausible statement which serves to back up and sustain the statement boldly expressed.

The experienced suggestionist has also learned the danger of attempting to logically prove by elaborate argument the statements of his suggestions. He also knows that when he has been foolish enough to follow this course of action the attention of the patient has been taken off the statement and the suggestion and the suggestion loses its effect. Realizing that suggestion enters the back door of the mind while reason and logic enters the front door. Suggestion is not based upon logic or reason. When a suggestion awakens desirable feelings, emotions or pictures in the mind of the patient, then the patient requires a small amount of proof or reasoning to satisfy their mind. People generally want excuses for their feelings not reasons or logical proof. They want to believe that which appeals to their desires and feelings. Therefore a small amount of proof is plausible "reason" to satisfy them fully, while an elaborate attempt at logical proof distracts their attention and causes the statement of the suggestion to lose its effect.

It is for this reason that Mental Suggestion is so powerful in Mental Healing. The mind of the patient is filled with the desire to be cured and have health restored. This being the case, the entire emotional nature is strongly alive to suggestions of cure. There is no opposition to suggestions of cure and health, but there is eagerness to accept any plausible reason or explanation of the way in which the cure is to be affected. The emotional nature is willing and eager to cooperate with the statement of health and cure rather than to oppose it. When you add a strong mental command, bold statement and authoritative statement of the suggestion properly made, we have a most effective and efficient piece of mental machinery set into operation and motion.

There are three strong mental factors operating in the case of Mental Suggestion when properly applied:

(1) Earnest Attention
(2) Expectant Attention
(3) Pleasurable Mental States

Let us consider each of these, for their importance must not be over looked.

(1) **Earnest Attention.** The effect of any suggestion depends upon the degree of attention given to it. This arises from the well-known psychological principle that the degree of perceptive impression of a sensation, the degree of its retention in the subconscious memory, and the degree of ease of the recollection of the memory depending upon the degree of attention given to it. Attention has been compared to the focus of a telescope. The strength of all mental impressions depends upon the degree of attention given at the time of their reception. The reason certain impressions stand out in our minds is based on the amount of concentrated attention that was manifested at the time the impression was received. If we gave no attention at all to an object of happening in the world outside of our mind we would receive no impression at all regarding it. This is one of the fundamental facts of psychology, remember it.

The patient coming to the Mental Healer for treatment is filled with interest and curiosity regarding the healer and their methods. The patient is like a child visiting a new place of interest and his mind is open to even the slightest impression and he is in a mental state most favorable to suggestion. In fact, the patient is in a condition in which suggestion has an exaggerated effect. It's very important the practitioner create a strong initial impression, by manner, demeanor and words, before, during and after the suggestive treatment.

(2) **Expectant Attention**. Practical psychologists recognize the value of the mental state known as Expectant Attention. It is an established fact that the expectancy, or hope, of an improvement in the physical condition will act powerfully in the direction of inducing the desired condition. This is the secret of the power of Faith and Hope in all Mental Healing. The secret of the cures of Faith Healers and religious healing cults. But, it may be argued, the average patient has not much faith or hope when he visits a Mental Healer for the first time. This is a mistake, the patient would not be there if they didn't have some kind of faith and hope for the outcome. Although the patient may say they have no hope or faith in the treatment, the very fact that they considered such treatment, went to see the practitioner, and paid the fee for treatment is proof that faith and hope abide within their mind. The spark is there and it is for the practitioner to blow it up into a flame; for it is a mental state which acts powerfully in the direction of a cure.

(3) **Pleasurable Mental States**. Another principle of psychological healing is that of a pleasurable mental state. It is conductive to the cure of the disease, while the reverse condition tends to induce imperfect and abnormal physiological action. Worry and Fear are potent causes of disease. Fearlessness and Cheerfulness are potent causes of cure and restored health. The practitioner should always "cheer up" and encourage the patient's feelings as an important part of treatment. The very encouragement of Faith and Hope in itself tends to produce pleasurable feelings and

emotions in the patient and the effect of the suggestive treatment. A skillful practitioner of Mental Suggestion manages to work in many little suggestions of cheerfulness and happiness along with healing suggestions. Sending your patient out the door with a strong suggestion of "You are Bright, Cheerful, Happy, Strong and Well!" the very repetition of positive uplifting words to oneself tends to induce an uplifting emotion and feeling. The perfect effect for a patient whose mind is receptive to suggestion.

12 PRINCIPALS OF SUGGESTION

There are certain leading principles connected to the effective use of Mental Suggestion which should be carefully studied by the practitioner of Mental Healing. These principles are not concerned with the nature of Mental Suggestion itself, but rather with the application of it. Particularly in the work of Mental Healing. I shall direct your attention to each of these principles and I ask that you carefully make note of the spirit underlying each.

Authority. The principle of Authority is an important one in the application of Mental Suggestion. It is based upon the well-established psychological law that the mind of the average person is strongly impressed by statement, spoken or written words, which are expressed with the air of strong authority. It makes little or no difference whether the authority is real, or whether it is assumed, just as long as the air carries with it the assumption and implicit assertion of authority. This fact is well known to many students of human nature, especially to those whose success depends upon the acceptance of their statements or suggestions to the public.

It seems that the tacit assertion of authority on the part of someone posing as a leader of thought, or practitioner of law, medicine or theology, robs the average listener of his desire to analyze, weigh, consider and demand proof of the assertions made to him. In the same way there are found many persons who will question statements made to them in conversation, whereas they accept without question the same kind of statements made from the pulpit or printed in the pages of a book. There seems to be some power in the printed word, or word spoken from the pulpit or judges bench, to render unnecessary the production of proof of the truth of the word. The proof is taken for granted.

Some psychologists have compared this acceptance of suggestions and statements made with an air of authority to swallowing food whole instead of tasting and chewing it. No matter how you look at it the fact remains that a suggestion given with the air and in a manner of one having authority has a much greater effect than the same suggestion given with an air of "everydayness" or doubt. A strange but true fact of human psychology. The saying "thus said the Lord" manner, air and tone of the voice has carried home many suggestions and statements which has but little strength in itself. The powerful suggestor is he whose attitude, manner, demeanor, tone of voice, and general expression of appearance strongly proclaims "there is no doubt here!"

Some people will obey any authoritative tone and manner. They are most effective on those who have never used their own wits and resources in life, but who have depended upon others for orders and instructions. The degree of suggestibility along these lines of decreases as we ascend among people who have had to "do things" for themselves and who have not depended on others so much.

The practitioner of Mental Suggestion will do well to preserve a gravity of demeanor and manner, and to pursue positive tones of authority when giving suggestions. The tones must carry with them the impression that he believes thoroughly in the truth of what he is saying and that there is not even a shadow of a doubt that the desirable result will happen. There must always be the air of certainty, lack of doubt or indecision, and the tone of conviction. The patient is very receptive to such strong influences and likewise to those of an opposite or negative character.

Association. The principle of Association is also a very important one in Mental Suggestion, as well as in every other form of mental impression or mental process. The Law of Association makes it much easier for the persona to think of things in connection with other things, than to think of things by themselves. Self-analysis will show one that he is in the habit of judging things largely by reason of their association with certain other things. And, likewise, if these certain other things be present in connection with a third thing, then that third thing is identified with the first thing even though there be but little real sameness between them.

A suggestion is more likely to be successful if the idea is introduced by a person, who is trusted, loved or feared, or under circumstances that inspire these sentiments, or in a tone of voice or with a manner that one has always associated with ideas that are to be acted on or believed. One or the other of these qualities or a combination of them is an invariable characteristic of the person who is suggestive.

The practitioner of Mental Suggestion should take care to assume the general appearance, manner and surroundings which are associated in the mind of the patient with a successful physician. The patient associates healing of disease with certain mannerisms of the successful physician and if the practitioner gives him the same impression he will feel more certain of the result and of the virtue of the methods to be used.

Earnestness. Earnestness has a great suggestive value. The public speaker, preacher, or lawyer who manifests earnestness and belief in what he is saying has a decided advantage over those who fail to manifest the same suggestive principle. Earnestness and belief are more or less contagious. We are affected by these notes in the voices of those to whom we listen. The patient coming for suggestive treatment is quite sensitive to these vibrations and is strongly responsive to them. A few words uttered in an earnest, confident manner will accomplish far more than a long speech delivered in a manner that does not carry earnestness and the tone of confidence and belief.

The quality of voice counts for more than we suspect in the relations of daily life. The speaker's power to move us depends on their being able to create in us the feeling by which he is or pretends to be moved and that will cause similar vibrations in our own nervous system. In this respect we are like musical glasses. We ring when we are in unison with the exciting object but not otherwise. Only words that come from the heart can reach the heart. For this reason a speaker who speaks out of the fullness of his heart will be more suggestive, will create more nerve vibrations amongst his hearers than any other man who has the same amount of feeling but cannot convey what he feels in the same manner. The more one thinks of it, the more plainly it appears in all regions of thought, the pivot on which everything turns, what importance we attach to it colors our every idea on every subject. The personal is the one thing that interests us the most.

The student or practitioner of Mental Suggestion should never lose sight of the fact that earnestness in giving Suggestion makes up for many deficiencies and when added to other strong qualities it becomes almost irresistible. Cultivate the air, tones and vibrations of earnestness and half your battle is won. The earnest suggestor will "get over" even a poorly worded suggestion, whereas a suggestor lacking earnestness will be unable to impact power and dynamic force to even the most carefully expressed suggestion. Here, as in many things in life, earnestness will often carry one through when all else fails him. It is the one quality which may be said to be absolutely essential in all Mental Suggestion in the treatment of physical ills. Earnestness covers up and cures a multitude of deficiencies and shortcomings in suggestion as in many other phases of mental activity. Cultivate earnestness!

Repetition. The principle of Repetition is an important one in Mental Suggestion. **Suggestion gains force by repetition.** It is a psychological analogy to the well-known physical examples of the repeated taps of the hammer will drive the nail into the wood or the constant dripping of the water wears away the stone. Each repetition of a positive suggestion will tend to make a deeper impression upon the subconscious mind. The same suggestion repeated in different words and with different illustrations will serve to greatly strengthen the original induced idea.

We have examples and illustrations of this in our everyday lives. We often refuse to accept certain ideas when they are first presented to us but after a while the constant repetition of them overcomes our resistance and we end by accepting the once neglected idea. In fact after a time we actually come to think that we have **always** believed it. The constant repetition of "they say" can ruin or build up someone's reputation. Advertisers thoroughly understand this principle of psychology and make good use of it. The constantly repeated suggestion of *anything* has brought us around to it eventually. Or the repeated suggestion that "you will eventually use this kind; why not use it now?" has done the work for many of us.

There is a weakened resistance through repetition of the attack, the force of habit. We have heard certain things affirmed over and over again until we have come to accept them as facts even though we have no personal knowledge of or any logical proof regarding them.

A politician of national reputation once said "Proof? We don't need proof! Tell the public anything solemnly and authoritatively and repeat it often enough and you will never need to prove anything!"

The practitioner of Mental Suggestion should realize the value of repetition in administering therapeutic suggestion and should carefully study out plans of stating the same thing over and over again in many ways, forms and style of expression. Learn to drive the suggestion home with many taps to wear away the adverse mental auto suggestions of beliefs by the repeated dripping of the drops of positive ideas and suggestions.

13 THERAPEUTIC SUGGESTIONS

One of the first things that the student of Therapeutic Suggestion must learn is that you must reach the mind of the patient along the accustomed channels of thought communication. You must not insist upon creating and establishing new channels through which your suggestions may flow into the mind of the patient. The sane and sensible plan is to first ascertain just what channels are open to you for use in this connection and then use them as the means of getting your suggestions into the mind of the patient.

This will be vigorously disputed by those who have been taught to believe in the absolute truth of some particular metaphysical or theological theory of cure. Such persons will insist that the first thing necessary is to instill the Truth into the mind of the patient and then base the subsequent treatment upon this foundation of Truth. This is all very well for those who see "Truth" crystallized into the particular teachings and doctrines of their own particular school, cult or science but the matter takes on a different significance and meaning to those of us whose vision is sufficiently broad to grasp the fact that all of these schools, cults and sciences, through their respective practitioners, are making cures in about the same percentage of results. Each of them has its own particular theory or doctrine which it asserts as "Truth" and as the basis of cure. Those who have grasped this fact find it logical to assume that all of these theories, doctrines and principles are but forms of applying some general principle of healing which is higher than any of the particular conceptions yet common to all of them.

The scientific student of Mental Therapeutics soon discovers that all of the formulas, methods and wording of the various treatments of these schools, cults and sciences are but the capsules in which are contained the real healing agency. He sees undoubted proof of this idea in the fact stated above and that cures are made under all these theories and methods in about the same percentage. Once this point is grasped the practitioner proceeds to adapt his methods and suggestions to the particular requirements of each particular patient. He first discovers the mental and emotional characteristics of the patient and then proceeds to use these characteristics as channels through which his suggestive treatment may flow to the mind of the patient. He becomes "all things to all men" in the best meaning of this term. Taking the patient as he finds them, turns to the best qualities of the person as a whole considering all aspects including characteristic and idiosyncrasies. He then takes the material before him, just as it presents itself, and proceeds to work it over into what he desires it to be. He effectively applies the well-known principle of the "the law of least resistance."

Some may consider this an unworthy practice but the scientific mind does not regard it in that way. Science has no particular theological or metaphysical conception of Absolute Truth to which it seeks to convert all those coming for help, healing and health. It has no framework into which it must make all patients fit. So it stretches out the short ones and chops off the legs of the long ones, to make all conform and fit into the fixed dimensions of the Truth. Its only idea of Truth is Perfect Health. And it endeavors to develop a practical and actual manifestation of that Truth in the minds and bodies of the patients applying to it for help and cure. Instead of attempting to convert them to some particular metaphysical or theological theory.

A word of caution to those students and practitioners of Mental Healing: Do not attempt to preach this doctrine of

All-Truth to your patients, particularly when they first present themselves to you. First get them cured and well, and then you may give them practical instructions regarding the Law of Cure as may seem fit for them. Do not become a zealous dispeller of illusions regarding the theory and principles underlying Suggestive Therapeutics, for this is a great foolishness on your part. Your business is to make cures not to make converts. To teach health not doctrines or theories. It is a fact of human nature that most persons insist upon having their Truth well dressed in fancy trimmings and masks. The pure undiluted Truth has for them the alarming clearness of distilled water; they will miss the familiar taste and complain that it does not agree with them. The wise practitioner will ask "what flavor?" and then proceed to give mental medicine disguised with the preferred flavoring and coloring.

Is that hypocrisy? No. its common sense based on the experience with the race, and designed to produce the best results. "The end justifies the means." This plan is not the furthering of error but rather the transmutation of error into actual Truth, the Truth of perfect health. It is the Pragmatic Method as opposed to the Theoretical and Dogmatic Methods. Testing "Does it work out with good results?" or "Is it the Absolute Truth?" and then we ask "What is Truth?" until Absolute Truth is discovered. Then proceed along the lines of Working Truth, a Truth that works out with good results.

The practitioner of Mental Therapeutics will find that the patients who come to him for treatment may be grouped into the following general classes:

(1) Those who incline to the belief that Divine Power is the underlying principle of the cure
(2) Those who have dabbled somewhat in metaphysics and who favor some metaphysical explanation of the cure
(3) Those who are more or less familiar with the psychological principles really underlying the cure
(4) Those who are not much concerned with the

underlying principle but who would rather seek the cure just as they would seek electrical treatment, massage or even drug treatment.

The practitioner will do well to modify his treatment to fit the requirements of these different classes, which requirements he may easily ascertain by a skillful questioning of the patient at the first interview. A few leading questions will usually bring out the beliefs and opinions, the preferences and the prejudices of the patient. By following this rule the practitioner will not only make use of the deepest and wildest channel of suggestion but will also avoid antagonizing the patient by running contrary to his favorite theory and beliefs. Setting up an unnecessary and undesirable friction or resistance. By this I do not mean the practitioner should willfully deceive the patient or that he should play the hypocrite. This is not necessary or advisable, remember you're morals. Knowing the real principle employed, he may by a careful use of words in giving the suggestion practically surround his active principle with a pleasant capsule, and by doing this accomplish the best possible results for the patient.

The Religious Type – those that believe in Divine Power

The first class of patients, those that believe in Divine Power may be reminded that Divine Power is the back bone of all rational treatments. And that the treatment to be given is one of the many means which Divine Power has placed at the disposal of suffering humanity. The terms "Divine Love," "Power of the Spirit," and other phrases familiar to this class of patients will create the very best kind of mental atmosphere for them and will render them receptive to the healing suggestions. Religious emotion is a very powerful adjunct to suggestive treatment. Proven by the successes of those basing their healing upon the appeal to the religious feeling, faith and belief. This statement is based on Truth, even a skeptic or unbeliever will admit, so the practitioner is not deceiving the patient nor is he playing a hypocrite, in wording his suggestions along these lines.

The "Metaphysical" Type

This class of patients, the metaphysical type, will respond more readily to the suggestions in which the idea that the diseased condition results from "erroneous thought," or from a lack of perception of the fact that "All is Mind." The main idea to be brought out in such cases is that the physical condition is merely the reflection of the ideas and beliefs held in the mind. That the true and real mental state will result in the manifestation of a perfect physical condition. This is essentially true, although there is also a physical basis for the disease and the cure. Patients of this class are not interested in descriptions of the cells and organs of the body they prefer to regard these as unreal, while Mind is the sole reality. These people seem to have a great dislike for anything suggesting physiological facts and prefer to dwell in the thought of the Mind. Accordingly they must be reached in that way in order to receive benefit from treatment.

The "Psychological" Type

The psychological patients are open to scientific explanations of the cause and cure of disease. They will grasp the explanation of the cell minds and the organ minds and will absorb, assimilate and respond to suggestions given along those lines. While they will be repelled by the introduction of "religious talk" or metaphysics. Let them know just what you are seeking to accomplish and then proceed accordingly.

The "New Thing" Type

The "new thing" seekers require more or less mystery and

illusion in the treatment. They like to believe that the healer has some wonderful power of the mind which he is going to use for their benefit. Any plausible explanation will suffice in their case providing it is given in an authoritative manner with the tones of confident assurance and success. They seek the "strange, wonderful power" of the healer and the healer who carries out this idea is the one who will obtain the best results in such cases. These people like the words "psychic power" and "vital force" etc., and are impressed by strange terms and methods of administering the treatment. A scientific explanation will go over their heads and they will lose interest and accordingly will not get the best results. These people must be accepted as they are, not as they should be. The practitioner must take the raw material as he finds it and then work it over into better things. First, last and always his business is to make cures, rather than to teach and preach to these people.

14 WHAT TO SUGGEST TO PATIENTS

The first thing the practitioner should suggest to the patient is the fact that they are going to get better, and will eventually get well. The patient should be told the healing power is now under way and that the process will gain force as it precedes, each treatment adding a little further power to that of the previous sessions treatment.

In a dozen different ways and forms the patient should have induced in his mind the idea and mental picture of himself as restored to perfect health. An important feature of therapeutic suggestion is that the suggestion should paint the picture of the desired result. Bright pictures should be painted of the happiness, joy and general well-being which will be his when he finally acquires the desired result. And he should be led to look forward to that result each step of the way. His mind should be directed to the improvement which is to come as the result of the treatments. This stimulates the "expectant attention" and according to the well-established psychological law of healing, will tend to manifest in an actual physical condition.

It is especially helpful to paint the picture of a perfectly healthy person so that the patient gradually and unconsciously comes to hold in his mind the picture of himself as being just this kind of person. The physical body tends to gradually grow to be just like the ideal of himself as held in his mind. In fact the patient probably pulled himself down physically by holding thoughts and mental pictures of himself as diseased, weakened and looking wretchedly. Sick people are fond of looking in the mirror and commenting on how wretched they look physically. The more they do this the worse they get and the worse they get the more they look in the mirror and comment, creating an even worse mental image; and the worse mental image they create the worse they get. There is a vicious circle of mental and physical, physical and mental, cause and effect manifested here. By creating in the mind of the patient a new and better mental image and idea of himself the practitioner really starts into operation a "constructive circle" which works with as powerful an effect as the opposite kind mentioned.

But this is only the beginning of the suggestive treatment and should be blended with more specific and special suggestions. It is not enough that the patient be given general suggestions of health, although these alone are wonderfully effective and often work cures, the practitioner must also get down to the details of the case before him. He must find the cause of the problem and direct treatments at the cause.

In giving therapeutic suggestions, the practitioner will find it beneficial to hold in his mind that he talking directly to the Corporal Mind of the patient. He need not tell the patient this, for it would then turn into a long and technical explanation and discussion. Let the patient think that the practitioner means his ordinary everyday self when he says "you" in giving suggestions; but the practitioner should hold in his mind the idea and thought that when he says "you" (in the suggestive treatment) he is really addressing the Corporeal Mind. And he should also picture that Corporeal Mind as having a mentality something like that of an intelligent, bright and dutiful young child, with whom he knows. Strange as it may appear to those who know nothing about the inner explanation of the matter, it is fact that the Corporeal Mind will "make friends with" the practitioner who will open up friendly communication with it. At first a little shy, like the young child, it will become friendly and desirous of helping the practitioner in his work of healing.

This is a very strange fact of therapeutic psychology but it is one that every practitioner may ascertain for himself. And fortunate is the practitioner who is able to grasp the truth of this principle and who will apply it in actual practice.

Each and every organ of the body has its own distinct personality. The therapist may actually address his suggestions to the different organs by concentrating his attention upon them and using the word "you" in that sense when addressing his suggestions to the patient. There is no need to say anything about this to the patient, for reasons previously stated. The healer who holds in mind this idea that he is directly addressing the particular organ or part of the body is often able to reach into the very soul of that organ and persuade it to put forth its best energies in the work of cure.

Careful students and practitioners of Mental Healing have discovered that not only is there a personality in each organ mind but that also this personality varies according to the character of the work performed by the organ in question. For instance it has been discovered that the Liver is more or less stupid as compared with the other organs; it is heavy and dense mentally and needs to be spoken to sharply and sometimes even harshly, in order to get it to work properly. It is more like a pig than is any other organ of the body, and it needs to be treated accordingly.

The personality of the Heart is like that of a high-spirited, intelligent horse. The methods used on the Liver would not work on the Heart. The personality of the Stomach is like good natured, faithful dog. It has confidence in those it likes and when patiently taught, it's happy to obey to the best of its ability.

The way to reach the mind in the cells, cell groups, ganglia, organs, nerves, parts, etc., of the body is to address yourself directly to it just as you would to a person. You must think of the mind in the affected part as a person who is misbehaving. Direct it with authority, tell the cell mind what you expect of it, what is right for it to do, and it will obey. Every practitioner will make this knowledge his own and apply it in healing work; using many forms of disguising it if necessary. This knowledge produces wonderful effects when properly and intelligently applied.

15 THERAPEUTIC AUTO-SUGGESTIONS

The information in this lesson is designed to teach self-healing principles of Mental Healing as well as the healing of others by using the same principles.

Auto-Suggestion in general means the use of Mental Suggestion directed to one's own subconscious mind. In this form of Mental Suggestion the person enacts the dual role of suggestor and suggestee. They make the suggestions and receive the suggestions at the same time.

This may seem somewhat confusing at first but when the psychology of the process is analyzed you will notice it is natural and scientific just like all other forms of Mental Suggestion. The secret of the whole process is found in the fact that with Auto-Suggestion the conscious "I" suggests to the subconscious "Me." When you have grasped this concept you have gained the secret to all true Therapeutic Auto-Suggestion. And until you have fully grasped this fact, you will not be able to apply the principles of Therapeutic Auto-Suggestion effectively.

In order to get the best results of Therapeutic Auto-Suggestion you should make a clear mental distinction between the conscious self which is giving the suggestions and subconscious self which is receiving them. You should actually visualize the "I" suggesting and giving orders to the "Me." You should visualize the subconscious "Me" as a distinct entity, subordinate to the "I" and should give your suggestions in that spirit.

You should "talk to your self" as if you were speaking to another person. By doing this you will be able to register a much clearer, deeper and longer lasting impression. In making suggestions to yourself you should always address yourself as if you were speaking in third person. Example: instead of saying "I am courageous and fearless" you should suggest: "John Smith (use your name here) you are courageous and fearless, you fear nothing, every day you are gaining in courage and fearlessness and you are getting stronger and stronger every day you live." Do you get the idea? Try both methods now. Make a strong "I" affirmation and then try the "John Smith, you are, etc.," Imagine that you are addressing and suggesting to another person that you are building up and strengthening. You will find a new field of Auto-Suggestion opening up before you. A little knack is required, but a few tries will show you the value of these two methods. Talk to yourself as if you were an entirely different individual. Tell this person what you wish them to do and become, and how you expect them to act. You will be surprised to see how obedient the subconscious mentality will become. You will find that by using this method you will be able to just pour in the positive suggestions to your subconscious mind and that part of you will accept the impressions as if there were actually two persons taking part in the process. This is not child's play or make believe, it is a process based on sound psychological principles.

The principle of addressing the organ minds in suggestion has also been extended to Auto-Suggestion by the same authority, and those who have adopted these methods and principles of treatment. Addressing the mind in the organ having problems as if it were really an entity and directing suggestion directly to it is just as effective. It is also useful to tap the body directly over the location of the organ in question, using the tips of your fingers, to bring the cells in question to attention. This tapping seems to have a psychological effect in arousing and attracting the attention of the organ mind. After you tap, the talk that you give the organ will have a much greater effect.

Example: you are having trouble with your Liver, you should tap a little over the area where the Liver is located, and then tap a second time because the Liver is sometimes slow, stubborn and hard to arouse. Then have a chat with it and insist that it start working properly. This may seem foolish; but try it on a sluggish Liver and see how well it works. Of course, you should treat your Liver and your body right, and not impose unnatural tasks upon it by eating improperly. Treat it right and insist that it treats you right. You can often actually feel the Liver mind "getting busy" after a treatment like this.

In the case of the Stomach, if you treat the Stomach right and let it know that you have confidence in it and faith that it will perform its work of digesting your food properly. The trouble with many people is that they have abused their Stomachs so it has grown discouraged. Change your mental attitude towards your stomach and let it know. Feed it healthy foods and give it some love. You will notice how quickly it responds and how glad it is to do what you ask of it.

If you feel like any of your organs have "laid down on the job" reform yourself! And you will reform them. You will have to let them know the new state of affairs before they will take up new habits. Tell them that you expect them to operate at a certain time of the day and that you will faithfully attend to your part of the bargain by eating healthy and exercising. Keep this up until the new habit is firmly established.

Any principle that may be applied to the treatment of patient may also be applied by you in your own case, by means of Auto-Suggestion.

16 THOUGHT INDUCTION

The second and third general classes of Mental Healing methods are (a) Personal Thought Induction and (b) Distant Thought Induction. These two methods are based on the same general principle, that of the induction of healing thoughts by the practitioner into the subconscious mind of the patient. There are certain distinctions between the two methods which justify their classification as separate methods of application.

With Personal Thought Induction the practitioner is in the physical presence of the patient when the Mental Suggestion is given. The thoughts or ideas of the practitioner are radiated from his mind and are transformed into corresponding ideas or mental pictures in the mind of the patient.

The thoughts, ideas or mental pictures are held in the mind of the practitioner, and then radiated or transmitted to the mind of the patient, should be practically the same as those expressed in words by the suggestionist in Mental Suggestion. The practitioner should create in his own mind the thought, idea or mental picture of the same normal, healthy conditions which he seeks to suggest into the mind of the patient. He should see not only the patient as in good normal health, but also as having perfect healthy organs functioning naturally and efficiency. The clearness of this picture will determine the degree of success for the mental treatment.

And now for the scientific explanation of this method. Its impossible to give the ultimate explanation of this wonderful phenomenon – or any for that matter. Until we are able to state "what" it is and "how" it works. So I'm not going to even attempt to explain what Mind or Thought really is in its absolute nature. Instead I will try to explain how Mind or Thought works and manifests in the process of Thought Induction.

Definition of the term Induction as used in Physics: "The property or process by which one body having electrical or magnetic polarity produces it in another body without direct contact." A textbook on the subject informs us that "Electric induction is the action which electrified bodies exert at a distance on bodies in a natural state; Magnetic Induction is the action which magnetized bodies exert at a distance on bodies in a natural state." The same authority informs us that the technical meaning of the term "Induce" is to cause by proximity to it but without actual contact. An "Induced Current" is an electrical current developed in a conductor in proximity to, but not in contact with, other conductors traversed by intermittent or fluctuating currents; also, electric currents developed in conductors moving in the field of a magnet, or conductors within the field of a moving magnet. "Inductive Power" is the name given by Faraday to the property which bodies possess of transmitting the electric influence. To which comes within the field of induction of the first one. In fact, in such induction the electrical current is set up in a second conductor which is in proximity to, but not in contact with, a first conductor – the power is induced into the conductors without the necessity of a connecting conductor.

But, there is no proof that Thought radiates power in this way. Outside of the enormous mass of proof gathered by the various scientific societies investigating this class of phenomena, and that of private individuals working along the same line. There is however a scientific study that shows that all substances are radio-active and the proof that the brain is not only radio-active but that its activities register on

MRI's and other x-rays.

Above the scale of light vibrations visible to the human eye there are vast fields of light vibrations. In the field of the ultra-violet light rays many strange forms of chemical and other non-classified rays have been recorded.

So looking at electricity and magnetism we have a striking analogy of the process by which positive Thought induces in another mind similar Thought, providing the second mind comes within the "field of induction" or "field of influence" of the first mind. In the case of pure induction with electricity or magnetism there is no passage of an actual current traveling along the electric wire or other conductors; but rather a strange and unaccountable "stirring up" of power in the second object.

A process that is once chemical, physical and psychical goes on in the brain. A complex action of this kind is propagated through the gray matter, like waves are propagated in water. On the physiological side an idea is only a vibration, a vibration that is propagated, yet which does not exist. It is propagated as far as other vibrations allow. It is propagated more widely if it is felt on an emotional level yet it cannot go beyond a vibrational thought without being transformed. But, like force in general, it cannot remain in isolation, so it will escape in disguise.

A force that is transmitted meets other forces and if it is transformed only a little at a time usually limits itself to modifying another force at its own cost, without suffering. This is the case with forces that are persistent, concentrated and well insulated by their medium. This is the case with the physiological equilibrium, nerve force, psychic force, ideas, emotions and tendencies. These modify environment forces without themselves disappearing. They are imperceptibly transformed and, if the next man is of a nature exceptionally well adapted to them, they gain in inductive action.

The structure of the nervous substances, and the experiments preformed on the nerves and nerve centers establish beyond a doubt certain qualities as belonging to the brain. This force is of a current in nature, a power generated at one part of the structure is conveyed along an intervening substance and discharged at another part.

Most of us who are studying Mental Healing have satisfied ourselves with the fact of the phenomenon of Thought Induction. The above scientific statements are not offered as proof, but to give a practical working hypothesis to those whose minds require it in order to reason deductively from principle to manifestation.

17 THE PRACTICE OF THOUGHT INDUCTION

In giving treatments using Personal Thought Induction the practitioner should always keep in mind this one fundamental principle of practice: Thought Induction is silent Mental Suggestion.

You will need to practice in order to gain the confidence and ease, and get rid of the awkwardness that usually comes with the practice of an unfamiliar process. Rehearse in front of a mirror and/or record yourself so you may make adjustments to your manner when giving treatments of this kind.

Many practitioners who have taken this advice have gained great results. **Practice Exercise:** Stand before your mirror and treat your reflection as if it were another person. Begin by treating it for any complaint that a patient may present to you. You run no risk whatsoever by doing this – no danger of taking on a complaint – for your treatments are always constructive and uplifting, and never along the lines of diseased conditions. In practice, and in actual treatments, you should always hold the mental picture of the desired condition, not that of the diseased condition, and always make your silent suggestions along the lines of positive up-building, stating the conditions you wish to produce, and never which you wish to remove. Always point out the mental road you wish the Corporeal Mind to follow.

In practicing before the mirror, you should throw yourself into the exercise in full earnestness. Do not indulge in flippant and frivolous play regarding treatments. Do not merely think the idea of what you wish to silently suggest to the imaginary patient; but actually think the words in which you would express the idea if you were speaking to the patient. This formation of words in the mind and the projection of them in Thought Induction is very important. There is no magic in the words themselves but the action of the mind in crystallizing the idea into words gives concentrated force to them and they are projected with greatly increased power into the mind of the patient. When giving Thought Induction treatments remember to think in actual words. Form the actual words in your mind.

In these practice exercises and in giving actual treatments to patients while in their presence you should follow the same general rules which are then followed with giving an audible Mental Suggestion. You should throw the same degree of earnestness into the silent words that you would in the spoken words. You should encourage the same feeling of force and power within yourself, the same raising of your own vibrations so that they may become positive to those of the patient. You should remember the principle of Repetition and manage to repeat the same silent metal commands or suggestions a number of times.

Remember that you are actually and really addressing the Corporeal Mind of the patient in these silent treatments, just as truly as when you address the conscious mind of the person in an ordinary spoken course of instructions, commands or advice. The more you are able to realize this actual process the more force and power you will manifest. The subconscious mind is very quick to sense the degree of earnestness and belief, or the degree of lightness and unbelief in the mind of the practitioner. It is like a child or an intelligent animal, very keen to perceive shades of feeling or belief, truth or untruth.

In giving actual treatments by Personal Thought Induction you should instruct the patient to sit quietly in a comfortable position. Have a comfortable chair in your treating room for this purpose and keep your treating room as quiet and clean as possible. The lights should be dim or shaded, bright lights tend to distract the attention. The main theme of the treatment room should be of Quiet, Poise, Calm and Peace.

Ask the patient to sit quietly and easily, to relax himself completely, taking the tension off every muscle and every strain off the mind. You will be able to help him in this process by sitting quietly some little distance from him and placing yourself in the proper mental attitude. Sit quietly yourself, stilling your own feelings and thoughts, and you will gradually raise up your vibrations from the lower plane to that of Peace, Harmony and Heath. The patient will then sense these vibrations and will experience a feeling of Calmness and Peace. This stage is often marked by the patient giving a sign of relief and further relaxing of the mind and body.

With the desired mental condition having been produced in the patient, the practitioner should form a strong mental image or picture of the patient before him, presenting all the outward appearances of perfect health. He should see the patient as a strong, healthy, vigorous, happy man or woman. The practitioner should keep this idea or mental picture before him as much as possible during the entire treatment. He should refuse to think of or picture the patient in a condition of disease or weakness and should always insist upon his mind picturing the desired condition of health.

Then the practitioner should begin making the silent suggestions of the desired conditions, the conditions which he wishes to have manifested in the actual physical substance and form in the body of the patient. He should address the Corporeal Mind of the patient just as he would an actual entity. He may even address it as "Mind" just as he would a person and then tell "Mind" just what he wishes for the patient. He may likewise address the organ minds or cell minds of the body of the patient, just as he would do in Mental Suggestion or Auto-Suggestion. The principles of healing are the same, the difference are found in the forms of administering it.

The practitioner must take the mental position, that the physical body of the patient, in its entirety and in all its parts, down to even the cells composing it, is a moldable substance which may be molded by the thought influence and power of himself (the practitioner), just as the clay is molded by the hands of the potter or sculptor. The mental images and ideas projected from the mind of the practitioner, and the silent suggestions made by him in this form of treatment, are to be regarded as the tools of the potter or sculptor, and are to be used to shape and energize the patient as a whole. Under the silent force of the creative mind of the practitioner, the physical body of the patient must be thought of as being built-up, strengthened, and restored to normal functioning. All parts thought of as being built-up and energized, the cells thought of as doing their work with renewed energy and activity and the whole system flooded with vital force and energy. Vitality and life. Under the strong stimulus of thought, image and ideal held in the mind of the practitioner, the body of the patient should respond to the ideals of the practitioner, and should develop in strength, vigor and general health.

This same principle may be used by the person wishing to heal himself by means of Self-Treatment. What the mind of a healer can do for a patient, the mind of the patient can do for himself, providing he has the perseverance and persistence to carry out the principles of cure. The principle of Self-Healing by this method is precisely the same as that of the treatment of the patient by the practitioner.

In Self-Treatment the person should follow the methods and forms of treatment in Auto-Suggestion along with those described here. He should acquire the habit of thinking of his body as already being that which he wishes it to be.

The Corporeal Mind has the tendency to manifest into physical form the mental images concerning it which are habitually held in the mind of the person. This is no idle fantasy – it is a scientific fact. If the Corporeal Mind has followed after bad patterns, it is necessary for us to hold before it the pattern of the conditions which we wish it to manifest, if we wish to regain the normal natural condition.

And, the normal, natural condition of the body is TRUTH, and we are fully justified in insisting that the Corporeal Mind cast off the result of its imperfect and erroneous patterns. Adopting the perfect pattern of that which Nature intended us to be, that which is Truth. we have the right to insist the pattern of Truth be followed as a design, not that of error and untruth. This may sound somewhat metaphysical, but it is based upon the report of the great minds of the race, and we may demonstrate it by actual practice.

18 DISTANT THOUGHT INDUCTION

The third general class of methods used in the practice of Mental Healing is that known as Distant Thought Induction. In this form of treatment the thought vibrations of the practitioner are carried distances in space to the patient. It has been found that it is just as easy to treat a patient ten thousand miles away as it is one a hundred yards away.

In Distant Thought Induction the principle employed is precisely the same as that employed in Personal Thought Induction, plus the manifestation of certain mental activities which serve to carry the thought vibrations beyond the usual limits of Thought Induction.

The possibilities of Mental Healing are enormously increased by the discovery that Thought masters and annihilates space. The greater part of Mental healing is performed by this method. Some healers will not see patients in person but give all their treatments this way. They claim they can obtain far better results, by reason of the concentration possible only in this form of treatment and by the elimination of disturbing influences of the personal presence of the patient. This phase of Mental Healing is important, the student and practitioner should pay attention to its theory, principles and methods of application and manifestation.

There are those who while fully accepting and understanding the fact that Thought is radio-active, and that our mental vibrations surround us with a mental atmosphere, and that this mental atmosphere constitutes our field of mental induction which awakens similar vibrations in the minds of others coming within its influence, nevertheless find it difficult to accept the teachings that assert that Thought may be sent to a distance far from the sender, and there be received by the mind of another person.

I cannot understand why anyone should feel any doubt for the phenomenon known as Distance Healing. it is no more mysterious than the simplest case of mental induction when the two people are in personal contact, or in near proximity to each other. Example: Electricity. In electricity we have the transmission of the current over the wires, in Thought we have a similar transmission over the wires of the nervous system reaching to all parts of the body. In electricity we have the induction of a current without direct transmission, in Thought we have a similar induction of Thought without direct transmission. In electricity we have the transmission of a current, without the presence of wires, in Thought we have Distant Thought Induction or Telepathy at a distance. All of these phases of electricity are but forms of manifestation of one general principle and all these phases of Thought Induction are but forms of manifestation of one general principle. The analogy is one of those very striking instances of the operation of the Law of Correspondence in the phenomenal world.

One mind can act upon the another at a distance without the habitual medium of words, or any other visible means of communication. It appears unreasonable to reject this conclusion if we accept the facts. There is nothing unscientific in admitting that an idea can influence a brain from a distance. There can be no doubt that our physical force creates a movement of the ether, which transmits itself afar like all movements of ether, and becomes perceptible to brains in harmony with our own. The transformation of a psychic action into an ethereal movement, and the reverse, may be compared to what takes place in a telephone, where the receptive plate reconstructs the sonorous movement transmitted, not by means of sound, but by electricity.

Scientific authorities dwell almost altogether upon the action of the brain as a receiving instrument. They have overlooked the equally important, and equally true fact that the organ minds, the part minds, the cell minds and all the phases of the Corporeal Mind are capable of receiving the vibrations of the induced thought current, and of understanding them and of acting upon them. Were this not true, the phenomena of distant mental healing could not exist as it does today.

19 HOW OUR THOUGHTS TRAVEL

In practicing Distant Thought Induction, the practitioner should proceed along the same general lines of Personal Thought Induction. Remembering the mental attitude to be preserved, the character of the thoughts and mental pictures to be held in the mind and the character of silent mental suggestions, commands and instructions to be sent by the practitioner to the Corporeal Mind of the patient, or to his cells minds, organ minds, or parts minds. The only additional process necessary is the establishing of mental lines of communication between the practitioner and the mind of the patient.

Mental line building, using the familiar analogy of electricity. While it is true that in the case of the passage of the electric current over the telephone wire are employed, it is likewise true that in the case of electric induction the current does not pass over the conduction wires but rather leaps out of them and sets up a corresponding current in the neighboring conductor; likewise, in wireless telephones the current does not require wires to conduct it to its destination, but rather travels along ethereal lines of its own making until it reaches the receiving instrument which is attuned to it and which has attracted it. In precisely the same ways Thought proceeds to its destination – its three ways of proceeding almost perfectly corresponding to those of electricity. For instance, Thought travels over the wires of the nervous system and reaches each and every part of the body of its manifestor, setting them into activity and regulating their processes. Again, it leaps beyond the limits of the nervous system, and by induction sets up similar vibrations in the minds of those within its field of induction. And then it makes mental lines of its own over which it proceeds to a distance, where it sets up similar vibrations in the mind of the person to whom it is directed and who has attracted it.

In Distant Thought Induction the thought of the practitioner actually builds up its own lines of communication to the mind of the patient, and then travels over it. This may seem strange at first, for it's a natural question to ask "But how does it proceed at all when there are no lines or channels to carry it? How does it proceed to build its own lines and then travel over them? How does it get ahead of itself in order to build the lines over which it will travel on later?" these are legitimate and logical questions. And the answer is equally logical and natural: Thought projects from itself the lines over which it travels to a distance.

In the cases of both electric and thought currents, they both travel in all directions from the senders. So now you are probably wondering "How do we create this mind line?" and the answer is simple: You build the track, or mental path, by thinking about it. The simple process of Creative Thought itself performs the work of building the track, or laying down the line over which your thought vibrations shall travel. We do this unconsciously every day of our lives when we think of another person. Though in such cases there is seldom the degree of strength manifested which accompanies conscious deliberate efforts in this direction, there is usually lacking that concentration which produces forceful and effective results in the work of thought transmission.

The practitioner, in order to get the best results, should first establish a strong, clear, unobstructed line of mental communication with the patient; this will remain after treatment, and will make subsequent treatments easier. You should take care to keep the line in order, the track clear, by a little attention each day or so. This direct mental line or track is built by the practitioner simply by thinking it into existence, by visualizing it as in existence, by creating a mental picture of it as actually in existence. There is no need of going into metaphysical or occult explanation of this wonderful phenomenon.

The more vivid the practitioner can make this mental track or path between himself and the patient, the clearer he can visualize it in his "mind's eye," the more effective the current traveling over it will be. If he can instruct the patient to aid in this work of path building there will be a much greater connection existing between them, a mental agreement naturally always produces better results in these cases.

The practitioner will find that it will help him materially in this work of building up a mental path for the purpose of Distant Healing, if he forms a clear mental picture of the patient at a distance, and will direct his thought of track building toward him or her when he is establishing the connection. It is not necessary to visualize the actual appearance of the patient; it is sufficient that a general mental image of a person named So-and-So is seen in the distance and the mental track be built toward that person. It is an invariable rule of thought transmission, that the vibrations always travel over a path or track and that this track has to be built, consciously or unconsciously.

Occultists have for centuries been aware of the efficacy of that which has been called "The Astral Tube" in the process of distance thought transmission and the principle has been employed to advantage by many of the world's best distance healers, although others have preferred their own methods which in the end bring into effect the same general principles.

The Astral Tube. What occultists call the Astral Tube consists of the building up on the astral plane (part of your aura) a tube or tunnel which acts as a most effective channel for the transmission of thought currents or thought vibrations. It is created entirely by the creative power of the mind and depends for its strength and permanency upon the clearness and power of the visualization, or mental picturing, of the mind of the person creating it.

The Astral Tube is created by the person first shutting from his mind all disturbing influences and then concentrating upon the task of creating the image in the astral substance. He begins by gazing in the general direction of the person he wishes to build the tube on. Then he pictures in his mind a great cloud of smoke like substance filling the space between them. Then he mentally pierces that volume of astral vapor, by setting up a whirling motion in its center. Then he pictures this whirling motion proceeding like a miniature cyclone boring its way rapidly through the volume of smoke like substance and thus creating a tunnel like bore, tube, or circular opening through its entire extent, until finally appearing at the other end is perceived the figure of the person thought of. The subsequent opening up of this psychic channel is comparatively easy.

Remember that, in the words of the average person, this work is all in the imagination. The Creative Imagination, however, is not a thing of mere fancy but is a most powerful creative force on the astral plane. And astral plane phenomena are as real and actual as the phenomena of the material plane.

20 HOW TO HEAL WITH DISTANCE

In preparing the patient for your distant healing currents, he should be instructed to place himself in a receptive mental attitude toward such treatments. He should be taught to mentally open himself to the inflow of your healing thought current and to assume the mental attitude of perfect willingness to receive the flow. This removes the friction that subconscious mind sometimes has and makes your work much easier and more effective. **You should caution the patient against making himself receptive to all thought currents from the outside; he should be taught to make the mental statement that he is passive to your thoughts only, and resistive to all others which he does not wish to receive.**

Some patients like to be treated at a certain hour but it is not necessary for the success of the treatment. Many practitioners refuse to set or observe hours of treatment and instead give the treatment at times that are most convenient to them. The Corporeal Mind of the patient is always wide awake, always home, even when his conscious mind is wrapped in sleep. The patient may be informed of this and told all that is necessary is to take the general mental attitude that your healing thought currents are always welcome.

When the time for the treatment has arrived, you should strengthen and make clear the mental path or line which you have erected and firmly establish the connection. This you do by sitting quietly and thinking the line clear. A little practice and you will notice when the desired connection has been reached. You will notice a feeling of closeness to the patient – a strange sense of the two people being in the actual presence of each other. When you experience this feeling fully, then you will know that the conditions are favorable for the treatment. If you experience difficulty in securing these conditions, do not become worried, impatient or discouraged. A little calm concentration will bring about the desired result.

When you are satisfied that the best possible conditions have been secured and the best possible connection established, then you should proceed to visualize or mentally picture the patient as present in the same room with you. Forget about all the mental wires, paths, tracks or astral tubes (for the time being) for you have already established the connection and your thought process will subconsciously keep the line open until the treatment is complete. In imagination, see your patient as standing or seated before you (whichever you prefer). Throw yourself as thoroughly as possible into the idea of this direct presence. Do not waste time in trying to picture the features of the person, for indeed you may not know these. From this point proceed precisely as if you were giving the treatment of Mental Suggestion or Personal Thought Induction. **In every way act exactly as if he were actually in front of you in person.**

From this point, you are to proceed simply as you would in the case of a patient who had called upon you in person for treatment. Hold the same mental picture of the patient manifesting perfect health; give the same mental instructions to the Corporeal Mind, cell minds or organ minds, as you would in personal treatment by any method we have studied and considered. Address the person as if they are in front of you with "Good Morning" or "Good Afternoon" and end the session with "Goodbye". This may seem like fantastic nonsense but when you have tried it a few times you will see how naturally it comes to you and how effective it is. Do not dismiss anything contained in these lessons until you have given it a fair trial. All of these things are the result of actual experience of many of the world's best healers.

The following is a practical example of Distance Healing. The case is quite common and you will recognize it often. It is a general case of "run down health" arising from imperfect nutrition and poor elimination, which has resulted in weakness, poor blood supply, cold hands and feet, impaired sense of smell, hearing, and taste, poor memory, and dizziness in the head, etc. When you meet these cases in person, you recognize them by their appearance, and you will recognize the general symptoms when they tell you their troubles. Drug treatment does little or nothing for these patients and they soon develop into chronic cases. But the right kind of Mental Healing treatment soon works an improvement upon them, and if kept up nearly always results in a cure. You will notice that the treatment goes right to the spot, and is directed along the lines of scientific physiology plus scientific psychology.

Typical Case. Having established rapport between the patient and yourself, you create the mental picture or visualization of the patient as being actually present in the room with you. This being secured, you proceed to address the patient just as you would in the case of ordinary personal presence, "Good Morning Mrs. Smith! I'm glad to see you. You are looking good this morning – you know that you are going to get better, going to be perfectly well pretty soon, don't you? Of course you do! And that is just what is going to happen to you – you are going to get better at once and then still better and then better still and so on better and better each day, until in a short time we will have you all right again, enjoying better health than you ever did in your life. All you troubles gone and forgotten and you so happy and well and strong that you will seem like another woman. That is what this treatment is going to do for you, Mrs. Smith – and deep in your heart you realize it, do you not? Of course you do – you know it intuitively, and that's why you are here this morning; here to be cured and made well!"

"Mrs. Smith, I now see you as a strong, healthy woman. I see you before me as nature intended you to be, and as you really are in Truth. You have plumped out, your cheeks are rosy and lips red, your eyes are bright and your skin soft and pleasant to the touch. I can see into your body and there I perceive all of your organs functioning properly and busily engaged in their work of building up a strong and healthy body, and keeping it in that condition. Every part of your body is doing its work properly; every organ is functioning properly; every cell is doing its work splendidly, just as nature intended it to do. You have a strong, healthy body doing its work properly and that is why I see you before me as an ideal Healthy Woman. And, oh, how happy you seem to be well and strong once more."

"I see that your digestive organs are working splendidly, and are digesting and assimilating every bit of nourishment in the food you eat. Consequently, you have a good natural appetite for normal healthy food, even a crust of dry bread tastes good to you, for when you are chewing it you realize that you are extracting nourishment from it which is going to strengthen you and keep you strong. Your food is being transmuted into rich red blood which is coursing through your veins and building up every part of your body and strengthening it. Your brain is well nourished and this keeps your senses in good working order. You hear well, taste well, smell well, see well, and feel well – your sense organs are all working properly, because they are well nourished. Your hands and feet are warm, for there is plenty of blood going to them and nourishing them. Your head is clear and your memory is good, because your brain is now well nourished."

"Your organs of elimination are working beautifully, and are throwing out of the system all the waste matter and impurities that nature wishes to discard. Your bowels are working finely; you have a natural movement of the bowels once a day, at the time you set for it – and you always keep your engagement with your bowels, for you have promised to act well by them if they promise to act well by you, and you are both keeping your contract. Your reproductive organs are in perfect condition, and you have no trouble from them.

Your menstruation is regular and normal, and free from pain, for you have established a new order of things in your general care of the body, and all of the various parts and organs are responding properly."

"You are bright, cheerful and happy all the time, all the day, and everywhere. You take an interest in life, and see everywhere as a new and happy world. You take an interest in what is going on about you, and are keeping young and active. You feel the spirit of Youth bubbling in you, and you are enjoying Life anew."

Here you should give specific suggestion to the various organs of the body above referred to, or which may be reported as in trouble; you speak to them just as if they were separate entities. It makes no difference that the patient is distant in space from you, the principle is the same as if they were in front of you. In some cases you will get better results from the "general treatment" as above described; in others, you will get much better results from the organ mind or cell mind treatment. It is always better to try both in order to gain the benefit of both methods.

You should terminate the treatment with bidding the patient good-bye, and giving her a strong, hopeful suggestion or statement that she will find herself feeling better each hour, and that she will feel like another woman by the time of your next treatment. Remember, that all of your statements and suggestions reach the Corporeal Mind of the patient and the organ minds and cell minds as well. Like a little child listening quietly in a room, the Corporeal Mind of the patient is eagerly listening to every word of your treatment so be sure to get in the right kind of suggestions and statements, that they may take form in physical states and conditions.

21 PHYSIOLOGY OF MENTAL HEALING

All Mental healing is really the effect of the Mind or minds. Of the higher Mind over the minds in the organs, parts and cells of the body. when this fact and principle are grasped you will begin to realize that the work of healing must be directed to the cell minds and organ minds, either directly or else through the Corporeal Mind which is but the sum total of these subordinate minds. You will also realize that the most effective mental treatment must be along the lines of inducing normal activities in the organs and cells. While general appeal and course of energizing suggestions directed to the Corporeal Mind generally acts in the direction of cure, and is all that is needed. Scientific practice should include specific and special direction of the treatment to the particular organ, part, or cells which are manifesting problems.

You also grasp the idea that your treatment must not be along negative lines. That it must not consist of thoughts and words about the diseased conditions and that it should be expressly and invariably along positive and constructive lines. It must consist of thoughts and words about the normal, natural, healthy condition of the organ or part affected. The thought of the practitioner and his every word and suggestion must be along the lines of the condition he wishes to produce in the patient. He must always see and think of the desired condition as already existing.

But how is the practitioner to picture and treat for the normal, natural, healthy condition unless he knows just what these healthy, normal, natural conditions really are? The answer to this question is obvious. He cannot! So, a simple, plain, non-technical, clear presentation of the basic and fundamental fact of physiology – the facts of the natural and normal processes of the physical organs of a man or woman in the state of health – is needed.

We shall not dwell upon the diseased conditions of the parts or organs except in passing reference. This is entirely different from that of drug healing that keeps the minds and thoughts of people on the diseased condition and never on the healthy condition. Is it any wonder that so many physicians grow morbid on the subject of disease. Particularly the subject of the special class of diseases which they specialize in? in the view of what we know of the effect of mental images upon the physical states and conditions it is no wonder that so many of these disease specialists fall victim to their own favorite disease. It is also feared that in many cases of mental attitudes and mental images of these specialists actually induce corresponding diseased conditions in the bodies of the patients under their care. A simple understanding of the laws of mental suggestion show the reasonableness of this suspicion.

So we are pursuing an entirely opposite policy. Instead of following the method of the orthodox teachers of medicine who "stick to the old materialistic ideas and cultivate the thoughts engendered by close association with cadavers, morbid specimens, bacterial cultures, and pathology in general" I have adopted a plan of pointing out the Healthy, Natural, Normal Human Body. Holding this image in our minds as a pattern to be used in building up a like condition in the bodies of the patients. This may seem like a small thing to those who do not look beneath the superficial appearance of things but this is an important fact and one of great importance in the practice of Mental Healing.

Some people fail to recognize the great importance of the normal processes of that which we call "Nature" as manifested in the human body. Many have in a general way thought of Nature as merely a totality of mechanical forces, which operated by action and reaction, relation and interrelation, and general coordination, which caused the "happening" of the processes of the physical body. This is a grave error of judgment, and important results may depend upon its correction. If it were merely a question of philosophy or general belief I wouldn't bring it up. But as the success of the practitioner of Mental Healing depends materially upon his understanding of the activities underlying the processes of Nature, it is important that students of the subject be correctly informed regarding this.

Nature is not a totality of blind, lifeless forces. All Nature is alive and is permeated with Mind in every part. There is nothing lifeless or mindless in all of Nature. Without attempting to explain the almost inconceivable mystery of Nature's operations, I would like to positively assert the processes manifested in the physical body of every human being in a state of health show the presence of instinctive mind working toward the end of efficient work. The human body is the result of evolution, of efforts on the part of this instinctive mind to manifest better and still better results. Disease results from some interference with Nature's Laws. If Nature in the body can have her own way, unhindered by external forces, she will build up and maintain a perfectly healthy physical system, for her aim and ideal is always Perfect Health.

One thing that the practitioner may always count on in treatments is that Nature is always on his side in healing work. Nature has her twofold purpose (a) the preservation and well-being of the life of the individual and (b) the reproduction and survival of the species. She is constantly working toward those goals. When things interfere, she makes the best of it, and does the best she can in view of the imperfect material with which she has to work and the obstacles interfering with her full expression and manifestation. In the depths of the Corporeal Mind will be found this primitive and elementary urge of Nature toward Perfect Health. Something else to remember, Nature kills a man as well as bringing him to life. While man is in the limits of his natural years of life, Nature is always striving to keep him in health and strength. She intends that every part of man shall live out his normal period of time, and she intends that he shall live it in health and strength. If Nature's laws were not interfered with, disease and short-life would be just accidents.

Nature's work is always in the best interests of health and life, that even many conditions called "disease" are Nature's remedial processes. Nearly all acute disease is really a remedial process, when rightly understood. But when Nature is unable to accomplish her work, she apparently resigns herself to the task of making the best of it and struggles in a halting and limping fashion. This allows the diseased condition to become "chronic." In our treatments we really help Nature by imparting energy and activity to the cell minds and organ minds and this throws off the abnormal conditions. **All healing consists in restoring Nature's normal rule and operation.**

Nature in normal action maintains physical health and well-being. Any deviation from this normal standard of operations means ill-health or disease. The closer you study the conditions maintained by Nature when the body is in a state of Perfect Health, the better able you will be to direct your thought, suggestions and treatment.

General Directions for the following information:

(1) Carefully study the principles of Nature's operations as manifested in the particular area explained. Do not leave the lesson until you have formed a clear, general idea of the operations of Nature in that particular area and function. Go back to the subject over and over again until you have mastered it completely. It may help you in your study if you take notes and write a short synopsis of each area. Stick to it until you have a very clear idea of the subject in your mind; so clear that you may easily describe it to a friend in conversation.

(2) When you have gained a clear idea of the subject, you

should practice visualizing or forming a clear mental picture in your imagination of the process you have you have been studying. Try to picture it just as you would if you were actually viewing the process in a human body.

(3) When you come to practice, I want you to reproduce the idea and mental picture of this normal, natural, functioning of the organs in question, so that you may actually set up the processes in the body of the patient which will bring about just this kind of activity and normal functioning. Do you get the point? By creating the correct mental pattern in your mind, and then reproducing it in connection with your thoughts of the patient's body, you tend to make the ideal pattern take on objective form and activity in the patient's system.

THE NUTRITIVE PROCESSES

First of all the important process of Nature in her work of building-up, repairing and sustaining the human body are the processes of Nutrition. The processes of Nutrition are those by which the normal condition of life and growth of the living organism is maintained and which operate in the direction of the living tissues of the body taking from the blood nourishing materials or substances required for their repair and the performance of their healthy functions.

You will note the following two facts: (1) that tissues take nourishing material or substance in order that they may keep in repair and perform their healthy function. This nourishment is food, and the products of food; (2) that this nourishment is taken from the blood. Here we have two great facts of physical life: (a) that the tissues require and take up FOOD and (b) that this food is obtained from the BLOOD, and the blood only. (By tissues physiologists mean the material and substance of the organs, muscles, etc., composing the physical body.) The next thing to understand (1) how this nourishment gets into the blood and (2) how it is extracted and taken from the blood by the tissues.

Let's begin at the beginning. The food of the human being,

composed of animal and vegetable substance, is taken into the mouth where it is broken up into bits to be more easily digested a little later on. But in the mouth we also find the first steps of digestion. There are located in the mouth six important glands known as the salivary glands; four of these are located under the tongue and jaw and two in the cheeks in front of the ears. These glands manufacture and give forth through numerous ducts a fluid substance called "saliva." Mixing with the food the saliva performs the chemical process of converting the starchy portion of the food into sugar or glucose, and thus performing the first stage of its assimilation into the system this chemical process is continued as the food passes down the gullet, but practically ceases when the stomach is reached. (In cases of indigestion, it is well to give some extra attention to the cells composing these glands, in your general treatment, for it often happens that they are more or less inactive.)

The stomach is the great chemical laboratory of the body, and in it are performed many important chemical processes in the direction of converting the food-mass into the ultimate form of nourishment in which it is taken up by the blood. In the stomach, is manufactured, by countless minute glands, that strong digestive fluid known as "the gastric juice." This juice is a very powerful chemical substance which acts as a solvent upon the nitrogenous portions of the food and also upon the sugar of glucose into which the starches of the food have been converted by the saliva. One of its most active ingredients is that known as pepsin, which is a powerful digestive agent. About one gallon of gastric juice is manufactured by the healthy stomach each twenty four hours. It is mixed up with the food very thoroughly by a peculiar churning motion of the stomach which tosses and kneads the food-mass so that the gastric juice is well mixed with every particle of it and able to perform its chemical processes.

If this work of digestion in the stomach is not performed for any reason, example: the stomach having been weakened by abuse and over work, or by placing into it too much indigestible stuff, then fermentation is apt to result, and the food-mass, instead of being properly digested is converted into a putrefying, rotting, yeasty mass, which instead of nourishing the blood practically poisons it. In such cases we have dyspepsia and other diseases resulting from imperfect digestion and assimilation. With those cases the stomach and its glands should be specifically treated by the practitioner, and encouraged to perform their work properly. The stomach is a very obedient organ as far as its mentality is concerned. By proper treatment it may be encouraged to resume normal and natural functioning; but the patient should be told to treat it properly in return. In treating the stomach, address yourself not only to it in itself, but also to the glands manufacturing the gastric juice. It is astonishing how these glands will respond to an earnest appeal, and will manufacture a sufficient amount of pepsin in it to do the work properly. Treatment of this kind just before a meal will often give the patient a keen appetite and will result in perfect digestion of that meal. The experiment is most interesting and instructive.

After the food-mass has been treated by and in the stomach as described, it is passed on and out of the stomach on the right hand side and enters into what is known as the Small Intestine. The Small Intestine is a long tube which is twenty to thirty feet in length, but which is ingeniously coiled upon itself as to occupy a small space in the body. This intestine must not be confused with the Colon or large intestine which carries away the refuse or garbage of the system to be discharged from the body. The Small Intestine is an important part of the main organs of nutrition. Its surface is lined with a velvety substance which brushes against the food-mass as it passes along and acts to absorb the fluid food-substance when properly digested.

When the food-mass enters the Small Intestine it is met with a strong fluid called Bile which becomes thoroughly mixed up with it and worked into it. The Bile is manufactured by the Liver to the extent of about two quarts a day and is stored up for future use in what is called the Gall-Bladder. There is also poured into the food in this stage a fluid called Pancreatic Juice, which is manufactured to the extent of about one and a half pints daily by the Pancreas, an organ located just behind the stomach. The work of the Bile and Pancreatic Juice is to act upon the fatty portions of the food-mass rendering it capable of being absorbed into the blood. The Bile also acts to prevent decomposition and putrefaction of the food as it passes through the intestine and also to neutralize the gastric juice which has already performed its work and is no longer needed by the system.

In cases of digestive trouble, the practitioner should always treat the Small Intestine, Pancreas and the Liver. The first two organs are quite receptive and responsive to mental treatment. The Liver is a little stubborn and must be treated vigorously, firmly, positively and emphatically told that it must get to work properly and efficiently.

The food-mass in the Small Intestine is a soft, semi liquid substance produced by the process of digestion of the food originally taken into the mouth. It reaches the Small Intestine from the stomach in the form of a pasty substance called Chyme. This Chyme is transferred by the intestinal juices and Bile into three substances: (1) Peptone, derived from the digestion of albuminous substances (2) Chyle, derived from the emulsion of the fatty substances and (3) Glucose, derived from the transformation of the starchy substances. It should be noted, that the fluids liberated from the solids in the process of digestion in the stomach do not reach the Small Intestine at all, instead they are rapidly taken up by the absorbent apparatus of the stomach and carried into the blood, then to the kidneys and bladder where they are voided from the system in the urine. Some of the fluids are retained in the body to perform necessary work.

The work of absorption of the digested food substances, or nourishment, from the Small Intestine into the blood is performed by the millions of plush-like hairs of the velvety inner surface of the Small Intestine, which maintain a constant waving motion through the semi-liquid digested food. They "lick-up" and absorb the nourishments now fitted for the system. In this way the Peptone and Glucose are carried into the blood to the Liver and then passed through the heart. The Chyle is absorbed by the lymphatic vessels called "the lacteals" and then to the thoracic duct, and then gradually conveyed to the blood.

In most cases of chronic ailments the original cause of the trouble is to be found in these main organs of nutrition. If the body is not sufficiently nourished, or if is furnished the improper material, it is bound to rebel and manifest in the form of abnormal function or disease. No matter what may be the superficial symptoms, it will always be well to take these organs into account and to give them proper treatment. If the body is properly nourished, and its waste products are properly carried off, the liability of disease is lessened and the work of cure is much easier and simpler.

The body has often been compared to a piece of intricate machinery, which is run by the steam of the vital force. This steam is generated by the fires of the furnace of the organs of nutrition and these fires must be kept well supplied with the proper kind of nourishment, the proper kind of food, and fanned by the draft of perfect functioning. Also, the work of the organs of elimination must be kept normal and in working order.

Two main points to keep in mind: attend well to the organs of nutrition and those of elimination and nine-tenths of your work is accomplished.

THE ELIMINATIVE PROCESSES

Second in importance of the body are its eliminative processes. No matter how well the body may be nourished it will not remain in a state of health if it is unable to eliminate properly its waste products, debris and garbage.

The word "eliminate" means: to put out, to expel, to discharge. The body eliminates its waste matter and products in four ways: (1) through the breath (2) through the skin, in perspiration (3) through the kidneys, in urine and (4) through the bowels, in feces or excrement.

Later we will go into more detail the process of elimination through the breath, in which the waste products of the system, carried in the blood to the lungs, are there consumed by the oxygen in the air breathed into the lungs and expelled in the form of carbonic acid gas.

Elimination through the skin by perspiration is a more important process than realized by the average person. There are over three million sweat glands in the human body, the combined length of the secreting tubes being about two or three miles. The normal adult human being excretes about one and a half pint to two pints of perspiration every twenty-four hours, that amount of course being greatly exceeded by people doing manual work in hot places. Sweat or perspiration is seen by chemical analysis to be loaded with the refuse matter of the system, there is very little difference between sweat and urine in its chemical composition. The excretory glands of the skin are really supplementary organs to the kidneys, and in the case of kidney troubles they perform a great deal of the work that ordinarily falls to the kidneys.

The kidneys are two organs located in the loins, behind the intestines, one on each side of the spinal column. They are shaped like a bean, and are about four inches long, two inches wide and one inch thick. Their function is to purify the blood by extracting from it a poisonous substance called urea, and certain other waste products of the system that would cause blood poisoning if not eliminated from the system. The watery fluid secreted by the kidneys is called urine and is carried from the kidneys to the bladder, where it is stored up to be voided from the body in the process of urination.

"The bowels" is a term commonly employed to indicate the Large Intestine, or Colon, into which the undigested food and discarded material of food is passed from the Small Intestine; and through which it passes in the process of elimination or excretion which ends in its discharge from the body in the act of evacuation, stool or movement. The Colon is a large tubular intestine nearly five feet in length, which passes up from the lower right hand side of abdomen then across the abdomen to the upper left hand side, then down along the left hand side to its lower portion where it makes a twist or curve and then grows smaller and ends in the rectum or exit from the system. Its termination being the anus or posterior opening through which the excrement is expelled in the "movement" or stool.

The Small Intestine empties its discarded matter into the colon by a curious little trapdoor arrangement on the lower right hand side of the abdomen – the Vermiform Appendix being situated just below this entrance. The waste matter of feces then rises slowly up the right hand side of the Colon; then along its horizontal length, which extends across the abdomen; then down the left hand side of the Colon, into the curve or twist called the Sigmoid Flexure, and then into the rectum, and finally out through the anus. Its movement along the length of the Colon is caused by certain muscular movements provided for that purpose.

The Colon is the great sewer of the system, which Nature has provided for the carrying off of waste products resulting from undigested or indigestible portions of food, and other waste products of the system. Nature intended that this sewerage should be removed speedily. But the artificial habits and customs of adult human beings has sadly interfered with this natural and normal custom and bad results have ensued for the race. But Nature accommodates herself to circumstances and if man would only carry out a settled plan of preparing for a movement of the bowels each day, and adhering to his resolve to give Nature a chance to do this work for him, he would manage to get along with practically no trouble in this area. But some will not even do this, they refuse to heed Nature's calls until Nature becomes discouraged and does as little as she can help – and the result is chronic constipation with all of its attendant evils.

Let's look at the results of this unnatural state of affairs. In the first place the inner walls of the Colon become incrusted with impacted fecal matter, some of it remaining there for many days, its fluids becoming absorbed until the remaining mass becomes quite hard and tightly packed together. A small hole is worked through this hardened mass, through which a small quantity of excrement is passed. The Colon so impacted and incrusted becomes a source of danger to the general system – it is like a choked up sewer flowing through a city. The fluid portion is absorbed into the blood through the walls of the intestine, and tends to poison the blood and all the parts of the body. This state of affairs is manifested by foul breath, strong perspiration and strong urine – these resulting from Nature's efforts to get rid of the foul matter by some other route. Dyspepsia, liver troubles, kidney troubles, rheumatism, nervousness and many other ailments arise from this state of affairs. Many cases of female trouble are caused by the pressure of the impacted Colon upon the generative organs, and the poisoning of the of the latter by reason of their nearness to the foul sewer of the Colon.

The practitioner will discover that when he removes the causes of constipation, and takes away the original cause of the troubles the symptoms of many of these diseases will disappear. In fact, many of the best practitioners now proceed to first treat all their patients for the imperfect elimination. By doing so they remove the original causes of the particular diseases for which the patient has come for treatment. The patient may easily determine whether or not his or her Colon is in this abnormal condition by the examination of the color of the stool. The waste matter of feces when first passed into the Colon from the small intestine is of a pasty consistency and a light color. If the bowels operate naturally the feces is discharged from the rectum in a soft state and of a light yellow color. The longer it remains in the Colon the darker it gets in color and the harder in consistency. Feces in a Colon which is very much incrusted often appears as a hard lump of a darker color. These facts make the diagnosis easy.

The practitioner will find that the Colon, as well as the kidneys, are quite receptive and amenable to suggestion, either given verbally or mentally. The Kidneys may be instructed to work more freely, or else refrain from excessive work as the case may be. The normal condition should always be the pattern held in mind and upon which the treatment is modelled. The Colon will respond quite readily to mental treatment having for its purpose the removal of Constipation. It will be found that the Colon actually seems to be fully aware of the existing state of affairs, and is anxious to have normal activity restored. But it has been so long neglected, and its calls and requests so persistently refused and denied, that it has lost interest, courage and activity, and has relapsed into a state of apathy. It has acquired bad habits and its cells and muscles have been weakened by disuse.

In treating Constipation, there are two things to remember: (1) the treatment of the Colon itself, you need to build it up so it may regain its normal natural energy. Also, you need to acquire the manifesting one movement a day, regularly and invariably. It must be thoroughly drilled and impressed with this idea, over and over again, until you have awakened in it its natural activities and have set into motion in it the vibrations which will raise it up to normal functioning. And (2) you must impress upon your patient (by word or letter) the importance of this condition being removed – the common sense of most patients will grasp the underlying theory of this matter as it is presented to them properly. The patient should be instructed to fix in mind a certain hour of the day when it will be most convenient to go to the bathroom and then to keep in mind that hour, and to regard it as a positive engagement. When the hour arrives the patient should retire to the bathroom in order to keep the engagement, even if he doesn't have the slightest call of Nature in that direction. This should be faithfully carried out each day, until the new habit has been fixed. This course will result in establishing the normal and natural habit of bowel evacuation. Your treatments should be along the same lines. That of normal, natural, regular habits of bowel evacuation. If you observe the above stated general principles and practice you should be able to cure cases of chronic constipation which have defied the efforts of the best drug practitioners.

In addition to the above methods of treating constipation you should encourage the patient to drink more water each day. The normal amount of water called for by our system is about two quarts in twenty-four hours on average. But very few people ever keep up to this standard – some fall far below it. Now, this is not advising your patient to take water as a remedy or medicine, any more than the use of food can be considered a remedy for malnutrition. The facts of the case are that unless the system is given sufficient fluids to work with it cannot carry on its processes naturally and normally. No matter how efficient its organs may be. Water is needed to absorb and carry off the waste products of the system in the blood, in the breath, in the perspiration, in the urine, and in the feces carried by the bowels. The mental healer should not attempt to ignore the plain facts of physiology in his enthusiasm regarding the Power of the Mind. Instead he should adapt his treatments to existing facts of physiology. He should fall in with Nature's ways instead of trying to run contrary to them. For in the end Nature performs the cures and Nature is the Corporeal Mind and its subordinate phases and forms.

THE BLOOD

In some mysterious way physical life and health is closely bound up with the blood supply and purity of it. It is amazing that the average person has but the slightest conception of the functions of the blood. The average man does not grasp the idea that the blood is filled with the nourishment extracted from the food and that the circulation of the blood is largely concerned with the distribution of this nourishment. Instead, he has a general hazy idea that the nourishment is "soaked up" by the system from the stomach in some unknown and mysterious way. He realizes that his blood is an important item of his physical well-being and that if it is weak or if he loses it he weakens or dies. But this is about as far as his thought of the subject extends.

I have found it advisable to inform patients of this because when they grasp the idea their minds seem to take up the suggestion more clearly and they unconsciously cooperate with the efforts of the practitioner to bring about improved nutrition of all parts of the body. the suggestion of "rich red blood, flowing to all parts of the body, building up and strengthening it, repairing and creating it anew," is one of greatest value in many cases. The patient easily and involuntarily makes a mental picture of the desired condition and applies it to his physical condition according to the rule that "mental ideas take form in physical conditions."

The blood is the red fluid which circulates through the arteries and veins of man and the higher animals. It is formed from the Chyle and Lymph when these substances are subjected to the action of the oxygen taken into the lungs by the process of inspiration. It is the general material from which all of the secretions of the body are derived. In the blood current is also carried away from the different parts of the body various noxious debris and waste products of the system, which are then carried to the crematory of the lungs to be burned up by the oxygen and then eliminated from the system in the form of carbonic-acid gas.

Blood has a salty taste and when fresh it has a peculiar odor. It is composed of about seventy-eight percent water, about six or seven percent albumen, about thirteen percent of coloring matter and a small percentage of fibrin, crystallizable fat, fluid fat and various mineral chemicals such as sodium and potassium chlorides, carbonates, phosphates, sulphates, and calcium and magnesium carbonates. Etc. under microscopic examination it is seen as a colorless liquid with many minute round red blood corpuscles floating in it and a smaller number of larger discs called "white blood cells" moving in the substance. The idea of the real nature of the blood may be grasped from the following statement "The blood is the immediate nourishment and sustenance of the tissues. Its composition is practically identical with that of the tissues; in fact, it is really liquid flesh."

The vessels which conduct the blood outward from the heart are known as Arteries and those which conduct it back to the heart are known as Veins. The blood in the arteries (called arterial blood) is a bright red color and the blood in the veins (called venous blood) is a dark, dull, blackish purple color. Arterial blood is highly charged with oxygen, venous blood is deoxidized or lacking in oxygen.

The nourishment of the food is taken into the blood by absorption from the organs of digestion. It reaches the heart and is then sent forward to all parts of the body in the current of rich, red arterial blood that has just been freshly oxygenated by the lungs. It is carried to all parts of the body, where it is eagerly consumed by the various tissues and by them is converted into new cell substance, and tissue substance, and built into flesh, muscle and tissue in general. The body needs this new material in order to replace that which has broken down and been discarded and also to repair the remaining tissue substance.

The blood returning to the heart in the condition of dark, dirty venous blood carries with it the garbage and debris of the system, the particles of broken down cells and tissue, and other impurities of the system. Which, if left in the system, would poison it. This debris is bound for the crematory of the lungs where it is burned up by the oxygen inspired in the act of breathing. It is then cast forth in the form of carbonic-acid.

The heart is a hollow, pear shaped organ about the size of an average clenched fist. It is situated on the left hand side of the body between the two lungs. It is divided into four compartments, of which the two upper are called auricles, and the two lower called ventricles. The auricles have veins opening into them and the ventricles have arteries arising from them.

The returning venous blood reaches the right auricle and when it is filled to capacity its walls contract and expel the blood through an opening into the right ventricle; this in turn contracts and forces the blood through the pulmonary artery into the lungs. After the processes of the lungs have been performed the blood is forced back into the left auricle of the heart, which in turns forces it into the left ventricle. The left ventricle then forces the blood out into arteries through the aorta (the largest artery of the system).

The arterial system carries forward the blood current, first through the main arteries and then through the divisions and subdivisions ending in the tiny hair-like capillaries which reach to every cell and cell group in the body. The blood then giving out nourishment as is needed at the moment and having transferred a tiny particle of oxygen to such points where needed, then starts on its return journey to the lungs, this time taking the route of the veins, for it is now venous blood, dark dull, lacking in oxygen, and filled with impurities. It starts back first through the capillaries of the venous system, then passing on to the smaller veins, and then to the larger, and then to the main veins which pour it into the right auricle, from which it is passed via the right ventricle and the pulmonary artery into the lungs, there to be purified and oxygenated.

To some it seems strange to include the lungs when considering the subject of the blood but the sole purpose of the lungs is the work of cleansing and oxygenating the blood – without this there would be no use for lungs at all. Yet so ignorant is the general person of the principles of physiology that the lungs seem utterly devoid of any connection with the blood, and from any function to be performed in the direction indicated. There is a great need for public instruction of this point – for knowledge here certainly spells H E A L T H to mankind.

The Lungs are two in number and are located in the upper part of the trunk of the body commonly called "the chest." They are separate from each other by the heart and its blood vessels and the larger air tubes. The trachea, or windpipe, conveys the inspired air into the lungs; at its lower end it divides into the bronchial tubes which enter the lungs. The bronchial tubes then divide and subdivide into smaller tubes, like the branches and twigs of a tree, until they terminate into tiny lobules, or oval sacs or bags. These lobules or air spaces in the lungs are very small and very numerous; it is estimated that there are many millions of them in each lung. It has been estimated that if these air cells of the lungs were spread out on a plane surface they would extend over an area of nearly fifteen thousand square feet.

These tiny air cells are enmeshed in an intricate network of tiny capillaries of the circulatory system, which are filled with venous blood just returned from the various parts of the system to the lungs to be purified and oxygenated. It is estimated that about 35,000 pints of blood pass through these capillaries each twenty-four hours, the blood corpuscles passing in single file through these tiny capillary canals, each being exposed to a tiny particle of air on each side of the canals.

When the blood corpuscle comes in contact with the air in the lungs the oxygen in the air penetrates the coating of the coverings and, coming into direct contact with the blood, oxygenation and a process of chemical combustion takes place. In this process the oxygen burns up the filthy waste matter in the venous blood and converts it into carbonic acid gas which is then thrown out of the lungs in the expiring breath. At the same time the blood takes up tiny particles of oxygen which it carries to all parts of the system, where it is used in certain important processes in connection with the cells and tissues, serving to strengthen and invigorate, renovate and repair, every cell and tissue. Arterial blood carries with it about twenty-five percent of pure oxygen.

Not only does the oxygen in the blood perform the above function mentioned but it also materially aids in certain processes of digestion which depends on proper oxygenation. The combustion arising from the contact of the oxygen with the waste substances also generates heat and equalizes the temperature of the body.

In addition to the system of blood-circulation, there is another very important system existing and operating in cooperation with the former. This secondary system is called the Lymphatic System. Lymph closely resembles Blood in its composition. It is composed of some of the ingredients of the blood which have exuded from the walls of the blood vessels, and also of some of the waste materials of the system that require attention. The lymphatic system attends to this repair work and also several other functions of the system. The renovated waste material is passed once more into the blood, there to be used in the system. The lymph circulates in thin, very delicate tubes, which are invisible to the unaided human eye. These lymphatic tubes empty into several of the large veins, the lymph mingling with the returning venous blood and reaching the lungs and heart in due course. Certain portions of the food nourishment reach the lymphatic system from the intestines and undergo certain transforming processes before entering the blood supply.

The blood in one's body constitutes one-tenth of the body weight. Of this amount about one quarter is distributed in the heart, lungs, large arteries and veins; about one-quarter in the liver; about one-quarter in the muscles; the remaining one-quarter being distributed among the other organs and tissues; the brain utilizing about one-fifth of the entire quantity of blood in the system.

The general health of a person depends materially upon his supply of blood being adequate, rich and sufficiently well oxygenated. The richness of the blood depends upon the work of the organs of nutrition; its oxygenation depends upon the work of the lungs; and its normal action upon the work of the heart and the arterial and venous system. All of these organs are amenable to mental treatment.

The lungs are quite receptive to mental treatment and respond by displaying greater strength and activity, particularly when aided by the cultivation of the habit of proper breathing, which most persons have lost. The heart and the arterial and venous systems respond readily to mental treatment. Strong, positive mental suggestion will increase the circulation to any one part to which the attention and treatment is directed. The action of the heart has been found to respond to properly directed suggestion. The heart is the most intelligent and sensitive of all the organs of the body. it responds to loving, careful suggestions and advice but must never be driven or abused.

THE REPRODUCTIVE SYSTEM

Nature has two principal ends (1) the preservation and maintenance of the body of the individual being, in health, vigor and normal functioning and (2) the perpetuation and preservation of the race. The first end is served as we have just considered; the second end is served by the processes of generation and reproduction. Self-preservation and the instinct of sex and parenthood – these two constitute Nature's primal and elementary instincts and she has built up and maintained an intricate and elaborate mechanism to serve her purposes in both of these instinctive processes.

The reproductive organism of the male human being is as follows: (1) the Penis (2) the Testes (3) the Prostate Gland (4) the Cowper's Glands (5) the Vesiculae Seminales. The following give a general idea of the characteristics and functions of each.

The Penis is the intermittent reproductive organ of the male. The organ by and through which the seminal fluid is conveys from the male to the female reproductive organ ism. This organ consists of erectile tissue arranged in three cylindrical compartments, each of which is surrounded by a fibrous sheath. It consists of several part which are called the roots, the body and the extremity or glans penis. It is also surrounded by vessels, nerves and skin.

The Testes, or testicles, are two glands which secrete the seminal fluid of the male. They are egg shaped and are suspended in the scrotum or pouch by means of the spermatic cords. A short, closely contracted scrotum is generally regarded as a sign of the health of the reproductive organism and of the general system. While an elongated, flabby scrotum is regarded as a sign of physical depression and lack of vigor. Nature protects the testes by six separate coverings, the two outer ones of which are the muscles and skin of the scrotum. The spermatic cord is composed of arteries, veins, lymphatics, nerves and the excretory ducts of the testes and extend from the internal abdominal ring to the back part of the testicles which it supports in the scrotum.

The Prostate Gland is a muscular gland located in front of the neck of the bladder and at the beginning of the urethra or canal which carries the urine from the bladder, and which in the male also carries the seminal fluid. This gland resembles a horse-chestnut in shape and size. It secretes a milky fluid which passes through the prostatic ducts into the prostatic portion of the urethra. In middle-aged men this organ sometimes becomes enlarged and troublesome but this condition may be removed by the proper treatment.

The Cowper's Glands are two small glands, about the size of peas, situated one on each side of the membraneous portion of the urethra, close above the bulb, each gland having an excretory opening into the bulbous portion of the urethra.

The Vesiculae Seminales, or seminal vesicles, are two small pouches lying between the rectum and the base of the bladder; they serve as reservoirs for the semen and also for another fluid which accompanies the semen in its discharge. It has two ejaculatory ducts, one on each side.

The Semen, or seminal fluid is secreted by the testes and stored in the reservoirs of the vesiculae seminales. It consists of a colorless transparent fluid that contains solid particles of protoplasm, namely the seminal granules and the spermatozoa. Under sexual excitement the semen is forced from the vesiculae seminales by muscular contraction, and, passing into the urethra is met by the secretions of the Cowper's Glands and those of certain mucous follicles opening into the urethral passages; peristaltic action finally ejaculating the seminal fluid from the male organism. The spermatozoa are the essential element of the seminal fluid, the other fluids and secretions being merely accessory and secondary in function.

The Spermatozoa, or male elements of reproduction, are microscopic living creatures, each resembling a minute tadpole, with head, rod-like body and a hair like tail which is in constant motion from side to side. The tail serving to propel the creature to its destination. In the male human being the spermatozoa each measure about one six-hundredth of an inch in length and are present in countless numbers in the semen. They dwell in the gelatinous mass which composes a part of the seminal fluid of the male. The spermatozoa constitute the so-called "seed" of the male which impregnates the ovum of the female.

The reproductive organism of the female human being is grouped into two classes. The external organs and the internal organs.

The external reproductive organism of the female human being is as follows: (1) The Mons Veneris, or fatty eminence in front of the pubis, above the other external organs (2) the Labia Majora and the Labia Minora, the large and small liplike coverings enclosing and protecting the vaginal orifice (3) the Clitoris, a small organ hidden by the labia minora, having at its extremity a small sensitive tubercle (4) the Meatus Urinarius, or orifice of the urethra of the female, which lies near the vagina and about an inch below the clitoris – this is not a reproductive organ although associated with such. Its purpose is that of serving as a passage for the urine (5) the Vaginal Orifice, the outer entrance to the vagina and is located just below the meatus urinarius. It is surrounded by the sphincter vagina muscle.

The internal reproductive organism of the human female is composed of the following organs: (1) The Vagina, a canal or channel leading from the vaginal orifice to the uterus or womb which is situated in front of the rectum and behind the bladder. It extends in an upward and backward curve of about six inches in length and reaches and encloses the lower part of the neck of the uterus or womb. On either side of the vagina, near the orifice, are the two glands of Bartholine, which correspond closely to the Cowper's glands of the male, with excretory ducts opening upon the side of the labia minora. The vagina is lined with a muscular coat, a layer of erectile tissue, and an internal mucous lining. It is capable of great distension in childbirth, after which it resumes its normal dimensions. The purpose of the vagina is to serve as a channel for the introduction of the male seminal fluid; to sustain the weight of the uterus; to serve as a passage for the menstrual fluid and to afford a passage for the delivery of the infant at childbirth.

(2) The Uterus or womb is a hollow pear shaped muscular organ, about three inches long, two inches broad and one inch thick. It is the organ of gestation which receives the fecundated ovum in it cavity and supports and retains the fetus during its development. The upper and broader part is called the fundus; the lower contracted portion being called the cervix, or neck, which projects into the vagina. The uterus is composed of a muscular coat which contracts as do the walls of the stomach and bladder; this coat extends very greatly during the period of pregnancy. The uterus is located just behind and slightly above the bladder and is supported

by eight ligaments which, when in a healthy condition. Hold it firmly and easily in place. Displacement of the uterus is caused by the weakening or relaxing of some of these ligaments – this condition may be relieved and cured by proper treatment in the direction of strengthening the ligaments by suggestions directed to that area.

(3) The Fallopian Tubes are the ducts of the ovaries which serve to convey the ova from the ovaries to the cavity in the uterus; they are two in number, one on each side, each tube about four inches in length. They extend from either side of the fundus of the womb until they communicate with the ovaries.

(4) The Ovaries are two oval shaped organs lying one on each side of the uterus; the ova are formed in them, and they correspond to the testes in the male. They are about one and a half inches long, one inch wide and one half inch in thickness. They are covered with a dense, firm coating which encloses a soft fibrous tissue, abundantly supplied with blood vessels, which are called the stroma. Imbedded in the mesh like tissue of the stroma are numerous small, round transparent vesicles, in various stages of development, known as the Graafian follicles, which are lined with a layer of peculiar granular cells. These follicles are the receptacles or sacs which contain the ova or eggs, each vesicle containing a single ovum or egg.

(5) The Ovum, or egg, of the human female is a very small round body measuring from one two-hundred and fiftieth of an inch to one one-hundred-and-twentieth of an inch in diameter. It is surrounded with a transparent colorless envelope in which is contained the yolk consisting of globules of various sizes; the center of the yolk consisting of a thin transparent vesicle which in turn contains a tiny granular, opaque, yellow structure known as the germinal spot. This ovum, or egg, is discharged and enters the uterus at the menstrual period. When this period arrives the Graafian follicle becomes enlarged by reason of the accumulation of the fluids in its interior, and exerts such a steady and increasing pressure from within, outward, that the surrounding tissue yields with it and it finally protrudes

from the ovary and is then expelled from it with a gush. Following this rupture there occurs a hemorrhage from the vesicles of the follicle, the cavity being filled with blood which then coagulates and is retained in the Graafian follicle. The formation and development of the Graafian follicles begin at puberty and continues until the menopause or change of life in the woman. The ripening and discharge of the eggs produce a peculiar condition of congestion of the entire female generative organism, including the Fallopian tubes, uterus, vagina, etc.

Menstruation is the "monthly flow" of bloody fluid from the uterus which occurs in all healthy (but not pregnant) women from puberty until the menopause or "change of life." Puberty is the age at which a woman begins her period of possible child bearing. In temperate climates the average age if about fourteen years, while in tropical climates puberty occurs a year or two earlier and in artic zones a year or two later. The menopause or "change of life" in woman is the beginning of her period of non-reproduction. This time is reached when the woman is about forty-five years of age, on the average, although in some cases it is reached several years later and a few cases a little earlier. The general rule is that a woman's child bearing possibility extends over a period of thirty years, on average. At the time of menopause and after the ovaries diminish in size, the Graafian follicles cease to form and develop, the fallopian tubes atrophy and other physical changes manifest themselves.

Menstruation, when fully established, occurs at intervals of every twenty-eight days in healthy women; in some cases it occurs as often as every twenty-one days while in others is occurs as seldom as every six weeks, without effecting the general health or normal functioning. Menstruation ceases temporarily during pregnancy and also is inhibited during the period of nursing. The menstrual flow continues for about four or five says although there is a wide range of variation. The flow increases during the first part of the period and decreases during the last part. Menstruation is accompanied by the congestion previously noted and a sense of physical discomfort and irritable emotional feeling.

Menstruation is accompanied by a hypertrophy of the mucous membrane of the uterus, the shedding of this hypertrophied membrane leaves the underlying vessels exposed and bleeding. After the period new mucous membrane is formed. As stated before, the ovum is discharged and enters the uterus at this period.

The ovum, unless impregnated by a spermatozoon of the male, gradually loses its vitality and is thrown out of the system. If impregnated it remains attached to the walls of the uterus and in time develops into the fetus. The ovum contains all the rudiments of the young creature, but unless it is impregnated and fertilized by the sperm it never develops. The impregnated ovum begins to form a segmentation nucleus and then the segmentation or "splitting up" process begins and new cells rapidly form. There appears an opaque streak known as "the primitive trace" of the embryo, and the young living creature begins its life history. The period of gestation continues for about nine solar months, or about two hundred and eighty days, although in some cases it continues for only seven months and in other ten months.

The reproductive organism of both man and woman is very responsive to suggestion while in the womb and mental treatment along the lines indicated in these lessons. Weakened parts may be materially strengthened by the proper suggestions intelligently directed. In the case of weakness of the uterus, falling of the womb, etc., a line of suggestions directed toward the strengthening and contraction of the supporting ligaments and muscles will be found very effective. The uterus is very sensitive to mental treatment, and is much like the heart in its degree of intelligence and responsiveness. There is a great field for scientific mental treatment here and one in which medical science has failed to afford the best results – too often the surgeon's knife has been used needlessly. The skilled practitioner of mental healing who specializes in this area of cases should obtain wonderful results.

22 WHEN THE HAND OF THE POTTER SLIPS

In many oriental poems, such as "Rubaiyat" of Omar Khayyam, there is found a reference to the favorite oriental analogy of the Potter and the Pots – the Creative Power being the Potter and the human creature being the Pot which has been molded by the hand of the Potter. When a diseased or deformed body is seen it is then said "the hand of the Potter slipped." And this figurative picture is in close resemblance to the truth. for the hand of Nature at times does seem to "slip" in its work, although in many cases the slip is caused by an interference of the human creature with Nature's own well-laid plans and established machinery of operation. Nature being in this case merely the Corporeal Mind, it is seen that the slip is one of that wonderful mental organization and one which may be remedied by appealing directly to it.

The following is a general classification of ways in which "the hand of the Potter slips" so that the practitioner may see clearly the nature of the task of reparative work which he must impose upon the Corporeal Mind to perform so that the patient may regain health, strength and normal functioning. It is understood that the following is not a complete list of physical ailment, nor is it a lesson on pathology. It is merely a general classification, with general suggestion as to treatment of the "slips."

General Treatment

In most cases it will be found well for the practitioner to give the new patient a General Treatment. Example: a treatment for general health and strength. This is accomplished by treating each general function or activity of the body in turn, beginning with the main organs of nutrition then proceeding to the organs of elimination, then the organs of circulation, the heart, arteries and veins, etc., not forgetting the lungs in the connection. Then follow with the reproductive system, and then the muscles, joints, etc. In this way a general improvement of the whole system is started under way and a firm foundation is laid for subsequent special or local treatments for specific complaints. In many cases a General Treatment of the main organs of nutrition and elimination will cure the patient of his local and specific complaint. A patient in whom perfect nutrition and perfect elimination is effected generally manages to throw off the special complaint without much more trouble. The practitioner will do well to always keep this fact in mind, for it will explain many strange and rapid cures and will also give direction on the course of treatment in many puzzling cases which have defied other kinds of treatment.

Troubles of the Organs of Nutrition

The chief troubles in this area is malnutrition and dyspepsia, indigestion, etc. These problems usually are associated and existing at the same time. The course of treatment here is obvious. Treatment should be directed toward energizing the stomach and intestines into activity and normal functioning. The stomach should be urged to perform its work properly and the patient should be instructed to furnish it with wholesome food only. The small intestine should be urged to resume normal functioning and to aid in the work of digestion and assimilation in order that there may be created rich nourishing blood which will build up the entire system. The stomach of a dyspeptic is generally found to be in a state of panic, this must be relieved by proper suggestion and confidence restored. The stomach and intestines are quite intelligent and will respond quickly to the right kind of suggestion.

The liver is a slow stubborn organ and requires the most vigorous and positive kind of suggestions, orders, commands and general "scolding" in order to be made to resume normal functioning. It must be approached in a positive mental attitude – mastery must be asserted and maintained. A little actual practice will show the practitioner the best line of suggestions and commands to use in such cases but the general rule is to be firm and positive in dealing with the liver.

Troubles of the Organs of Elimination

The bowels, kidneys, and bladder are quiet receptive to suggestion and will respond to and cooperate with the efforts of the practitioner who approaches them in the right spirit and manner. There is but one general rule, and that is to tell the organ plainly and kindly just what is required of it and how it must behave itself. Train it just as you would an intelligent dog. You will be surprised at first to see how rapidly and intelligently the organ will respond. In the case of constipation, the patient should be instructed to make and keep his or her engagement with the bowels each day. To set a time and go to the bathroom whether or not an inclination is felt. The bowels will quickly respond to this confidence and will be felt to be actually and earnestly endeavoring to keep its part of the agreement. Where purgative medicines have been employed and the pill habit established it will take a longer time then otherwise to neutralize this old habit and to establish the new and normal one. Tendency to urinate to often may be checked by the proper suggestions and the muscles controlling the bladder may be taught to contract tighter and to maintain the contraction better and longer. The words tighten or loosen respectively convey a strong suggestion to this class of muscles. The sphincter muscles which surround, and by contraction tend to close, the various openings of the organs of elimination. In treating diarrhea and loose bowels, simply reverse the suggestions given in the case of constipation.

Troubles of the Heart and Circulation
The heart, and the arteries and veins, are very amenable to suggestion and will respond very intelligently to it when properly given. The heart is very gentle and intelligent and should be treated accordingly. Rough methods of treatment should be avoided in treating the heart or circulatory system in general; gentle, kind, soothing words and tones, and clear, plain, intelligent directions should be given to it. You may even explain to the heart the trouble that is being caused by imperfect action, accompanying as to how the trouble may be overcome, and new and better habits of action acquired. In case of cold hands or feet, you may direct and increased circulation to those parts by calling the attention of the circulatory system mind to the matter. Anemia, or deficient blood supply, is of course to be treated by improving the nutrition; for the heart cannot furnish nourishment to the blood, nor the blood to the parts of the body, unless it has been assimilated and absorbed from the food eaten by the patient. Dropsy, or an abnormal accumulation of serum, which causes swelling, etc., may be treated by stimulating the kidneys and the skin to carry off the excess fluids, and to thereafter perform their functions normally.

Troubles of the Lungs
The lungs respond very well to suggestions properly directed. The suggestion should be along the lines of increased activity and resistance. The cells should be urged to greater efforts, and taught to resist invading organisms. In cases of this kind, you should pay attention to the organs of nutrition also, for it is a fact that a well-nourished body is better able to fight off and defeat attacking organisms. The patient should be taught the value of correct breathing for the exercise of the lungs is often sufficient to prevent or to overcome weakness.

Rheumatic Troubles
Rheumatism is a condition arising from imperfect circulation and imperfect elimination. By treating both of these

conditions the special trouble tends to disappear.

Troubles of the Sense Organs

Weakness of sight, hearing, or smell may be treated by building up the general system, by providing proper nutrition and elimination and also by special energizing treatment directed to the core of the trouble. The cells may be energized into more normal functioning by an appeal directed immediately to them. The patient may aid materially such treatment by directing his or her attention to the organ in question and maintaining a mental attitude of expectant attention. This use of the mind of the patient, encouraged and supplemented by that of your own mind, will often bring marked and rapid results. Sense organs are very responsive to increased demands made upon them by their owner, particularly if the owner manifests a mental state of confident expectation – the organ seems to realize that better work is expected of it and it tries to "make good"; reversing the rule, the organ seems to realize distrust and lack of confidence in it and responds in like measure.

Neuralgic Troubles

Neuralgic troubles, headaches, etc., usually arise from imperfect nutrition, or imperfect elimination, or both, although in some cases these are found to be a condition of imperfect circulation. The treatment is obvious, when cause is perceived. The direction of the mind and the suggestions to the local parts however often relieve the immediate distress; but the healer should never be satisfied until he has removed the root of the trouble as well as the local symptoms.

Reproductive Complaints

The troubles of the male and female reproductive organism may be effectively treated by suggestion and mental treatment scientifically and intelligently applied. In the case of weakness of the male reproductive organism, mental treatment may be applied in the direction of a general energizing of the whole system, which is far more simple than the cases of women. In cases of weakness of the male, treatment may also be effectively directed to the lower part of the spinal column, where the bony parts spread out into a broad flat bone; for certain nerves in the region are closely connected with the male reproductive system.

In the case of weakness of the female reproduction system, suggestion and mental treatment is usually found very effective. Displacements of the uterus, falling of the womb, etc., are treated by suggestions to the supporting ligaments and muscles, and orders to them to contract and do better work in the direction of supporting the uterus properly. These ligaments respond very readily in most cases, and a marked improvement is speedily manifested. The general suggestion in such cases should be based on the mental pattern conveyed by the ideas "up" and "firmly in place." Menstrual troubles may be effectively treated by suggestions directed to the ovaries and uterus and to the reproductive system in general, the general thought being "normal and natural action." A heavy menses flow should be treated in the same way as diarrhea by suggestion of "slow" and "not so free" etc. In all cases of female troubles it is best to build up the general system, particularly the organs of nutrition and elimination. Many cases of uterine troubles originally arise from the presence of a distended, impacted colon. This condition resulting from constipation etc. When the cause is removed, it is a comparatively simple matter to remedy the local trouble.

Nervous Troubles

What are generally known as "nervous" troubles may be treated by first attending to the organs of nutrition and elimination and then by a special treatment of the spinal column. In the latter the thought must be swept up and down the spinal column, with the idea held in mind that the spinal column is being energized, freed from obstructing influences, conditions and tendencies. It is a good plan to finish any kind of treatment in this way – the sweeping of the spine acting as a general stimulating influence which is very gratifying and pleasant to the patient.

Another general treatment effective in all cases is that known as "equalizing the circulation" in which the thought sweeps down and then up over the whole body, several times in succession; this tends to energize and equalize the circulation over the entire system, bringing a pleasant tingling to the body of the patient, and resulting in a refreshing sensation and feeling afterwards.

Self-Treatment

The student who wishes to heal him or herself by means of Mental Healing has to remember that each and every form, method, principle and rule of treatment given in these lessons for the treatment of the patient is equally valid and applicable in the treatment of oneself. Apply the same treatment, in the same way, and you will obtain the same result in self-healing. the principle is identical and the methods of application are practically the same.

In Self-Treatment the "I" part of yourself should act as the practitioner, while the Corporeal Mind of yourself should be the patient. Proceed in such case as if you were really treating another person, the body of another. This is the whole secret in a few words.

Concluding Advice

In all forms of mental treatment, no matter what particular methods you may use, or what particular trouble you may be treating, you should always carry in mind the fact that THOUGHT is the active principle involved in the cure. And you should learn to think of Thought not as an intangible, unsubstantial thing, but rather as a great natural energy and force, something as real as electricity or magnetism. It will help you to mentally view it as sweeping from you into the body of the patient, there energizing and strengthening the minds in the cells and parts of the body. the more clearly that you can visualize or mentally picture it as actually traveling and moving like a great current of electricity, the greater its potency will be.

Do not allow yourself to be become wrapped up in

technical theories or speculations regarding the Riddle of the Universe, or of the inner nature of Mind. Leave these subjects to the meta-physicians who delight in them to such an extent that they usually have no time or inclination to do anything practical in life. Do not be a dreamer, but be a doer. Cultivate the characteristics of the Constructive Thinker – build up, construct, create, with the Power of the Mind. You will find that your Power to Heal will increase with practice and habit. You will develop what some have called "the sanative contagion," to such an extent that those coming into your presence will receive healing thought even though you do not voluntarily send it out. You will radiate healing power – this is the mark of the true healer. Think of yourself as a SUN of HEALING POWER and let your radiance flow in all directions.

You will learn new details of practice every year of your life; but you will always be impressed with the truth of the statement that the Principle of Mental Healing is very simple and plain when once grasped and understood. Here is a simple statement of this simple fact to carry with you always: **"Mental Patterns are reproduced in Physical States, Forms, and Conditions."**

ABOUT THE AUTHOR

Cindy Walker, Hypnotherapist & Essence of Life Healer

I have been called many things by many people. But my favorite is my title, Essence of Life Healer, it was given to me by the Entities of the Light whom I was working with while writing this guide book. I have many spiritual gift's and among them is the gift of channel. I was able to channel a few brilliant Entities that helped with the sharing of this information. We hope you enjoy it and that you are now able to heal yourself and others.